BORN A
CHAMPION

BORN A CHAMPION

The Master Strategy for
Maximum Health and Lasting Success

DR. DAVID YACHTER

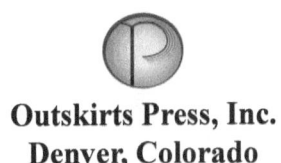

Outskirts Press, Inc.
Denver, Colorado

Outskirts Press, Inc.
http://www.outskirtspress.com

PB ISBN: 978-1-4327-4138-9
HB ISBN: 978-1-4327-4139-6

Outskirts Press and the "OP" logo are trademarks belonging to Outskirts Press, Inc.

PRINTED IN THE UNITED STATES OF AMERICA

"A Glorified body." I'll never forget the first time I heard that term. A huge smile was on the face of Ms. Fay Williams as she demonstrated her faith despite her amputated leg, multiple medical conditions, and wheelchair confinement. This woman was an angel placed in my life by God to teach me about faith, love, and courage. She was a very special patient indeed, many of whom reading this will remember very well. She was the first one in every morning, and the last one to leave. She loved to just sit in the office, greet, smile, silently pray for others, and watch their lives gradually transform. She unerringly had full 100% faith in God's law of healing from above- down, inside-out; dare I say more so than most doctors. Fay immersed herself in everything that had an opportunity to serve God by being an encouragement to others. She could be found at every workshop sitting in the back joyfully helping with registration. The next day she'd always say "Oh, Doc, yesterday's workshop was sooooooo good. It was the best one ever." Funny thing was, she said the same thing after every workshop- ALL 50 of them!

Fay passed away unexpectedly from complications, still yet unknown (although I do suspect hospital administrative errors). Her funeral was an absolute celebration of an amazing spirit of faith, triumph, and victory in God's ultimate commandment given to all mankind. Although I may not see her here anymore in the flesh, I will forever be reminded of her kind and sweet spirit of inspiration. She was not only my greatest fan, but more importantly, my greatest coach. In her loss, I have gained the realization of how much I need my patients as much as they need me.

Our encouragement, inspiration, and edification of one another is THE SINGLE MOST IMPORTANT ELEMENT necessary for change and transformation; not only for the one encouraged, but the encourager as well! Ironically, the best way to help one's self is to first help others. God's plan for you is to be a living example of this, in all you do.

If all I ever did was fix an individual's spine or pain, I should be considered a failure. My vision for you and your family goes way beyond that. With every word you read and every seminar you attend there are seeds of knowledge, wisdom, and greatness that are planted. Your continued learning cultivates seeds for a future harvest of abundant life, health, and longevity. Our goal is for you to live out all of your years; drug- free, maximum quality of life. However, success is not a goal or a destination, it is rather a journey. Along the journey, we are to reach out and take others along and show them the right path to life.

Thank you, Ms. Fay, for showing me the path. In doing so, you have exponentially helped me to reach out and save countless millions more lives. Our memories of you will truly be that of a glorified body!

Acknowledgements

To my wife Yvette: Thank you for keeping me on the straight and narrow path of life. Your gentle, loving spirit of truth is my anchor- the greatest gift that God has ever given me.

Thank you to my three boys:
Joshua; for your amazing heart and spirit of joy.
Leon; for your sense of strength, confidence, and certainty
Gavin; for your smile that brings happiness to us all

My brother Daniel: thank you for being an amazing champion, brother, friend, and leader in my life.

Mom and Dad: The early seeds planted did not return void! Thanks for never giving up on me and our family.

Dr. Sid Williams: Thank you for all you have done to defend our beloved profession. Giving me the Lasting Purpose of "Serving, Loving, and Giving out of unselfish abundant compassion" has radically transformed millions of lives exponentially through my own.

Contents

PART 3: FAT-BURNING FITNESS- conditioning your body for full time fat-burning.

PART 4: HOUSTON CONTROL

Preface

Outrageous Health. What a concept. What a feeling. What a blessing! In all my years as a practicing physician, I've never met anyone who said they wouldn't want to feel better, have more energy, and live longer. For something that seems like a no- brainer, why is it that there's more depression, disease, and early death these days than ever before? Great question. Simple answer: Lack of knowledge. It says in the Bible: "For lack of knowledge, my people perish." What was true thousands of years ago for Hosea, still stands true today. Some people know that they don't know, and even worse, others don't even know that they don't know. This book will be a journey into the wonders, secrets, and science of the mind, body, and spirit. All aspects of health, healing, and wellness will be discussed and discovered allowing you the opportunity to achieve your potential for optimal health and longevity.

Currently, the U.S. spends trillions of dollars on health care each year. While these expenditures for health are greater than any other country, we recently ranked almost worst in overall health relative to all other industrialized nations.* We have more cancer than any other country, with the death rate each year claiming 1 out of every 3 lives. Heart disease is also greatest in numbers here, claiming 1 out of every 2 lives each year. While the U.S. population consists of only 5% of the world's population, we consume more than 75% of all the prescription and over the counter drugs on planet Earth. With our country having the greatest technology, the best hospitals and doctors, and considered a world superpower, why is it that now more than ever we are witnessing the development of more illness and disease?

I want you to stop and think for a moment about your family members, friends, and co-workers. How many of them are suffering with or on medication for high blood pressure, cholesterol, cancer, diabetes, or depression? Without fail, when lecturing to large groups of people, a hands- up survey reveals about 80% are either personally affected or are affected by others that have these illnesses. Our families are sicker and more medicated than ever. There is more depression affecting adults, the numbers even greater in children, than ever. And the tragedy of it all? Medical research has shown time and time again that 70-85% of these diseases are treatable, preventable, and curable with proper lifestyle.

What is lifestyle? Exactly the way you treat your body, and the environment to which you subject it. In other words, it all comes down to what you think, what you eat, and how you breathe; working with the intelligence of the body instead of against it. Virtually 95% of a person's healing capacity comes from lifestyle, the other 5% is genetic "tendencies". I believe it matters less if heart disease or diabetes runs in your family, and matters more the way you steward your health with the choices you make. Remember rule # 1: God doesn't make junk. Whatever He created you with is built to go the distance. Science actually confirms that most cells in our body were constructed to last 125 years. So why is it that the end years for most folks are spent in a nursing home overmedicated, in diapers, being spoon-fed? Nearly always, this is attributable to side effects of prescription and over the counter drugs, hormonal imbalance, toxicity, and permanent impairment of the central nervous system.

The purpose of this book is that it becomes a tool for you to take care of yourself and your family for now and the generations to come. It will guard you from ignorance and help you avoid the deadly pitfalls of our current health care system. If you are disciplined and consistent in following the principles described in this book, you will undoubtedly achieve and sustain a level of health higher than you ever imagined possible. Now, let's begin building YOU a healthy future.

As a side note, many gems of wisdom found in this book are biblically inspired and have been of personal inspiration. Thus, I make no apologies for my contextual style of writing. Regardless of your religious affiliation or views, I believe the "true north" principles described in this book are practical and applicable for all who desire success in their health and life.

Part One

From Above-Down

Healthy Mind for a Healthy Body

CHAPTER 1

Discipline is Freedom

"Faith is the hostess that will not entertain doubt."
— Jenna Wright

Rule # 1: God doesn't make junk. If you were created in His image, then I believe you were born with everything needed to be healthy, joyful, and prosperous.

Rule # 2: Your body doesn't need any help it just needs NO INTERFERENCE.

If this makes sense, then all we need to do is not "mess up" God's perfect creation and Simply have a sensible plan for maintaining it. In the book of Corinthians it says "The body is the Temple of the Holy Spirit." Regaining and maintaining your health should begin with the mindset that your body does not belong to you, but the One who created you. It also says in 1Corinthians 6:20 to "Honor God with your body." Logically speaking, this would mean that having the obedience and discipline to live the healthy lifestyle that God created you for is a form of worship that glorifies God. Conversely, it can also be said that abusing your body with poor nutrition, lack of exercise, and destructive thoughts is dishonoring God. Thus, when we suffer from sickness and disease, we suffer from our own sinful nature. If this is sounding somewhat harsh, then consider the alternative. In times of crisis, everyone wants prayer and God's hand to intervene. But where is our relationship and discipline beforehand? Would you attempt to cheat God's law of gravity and jump off a 50 story building? Is it faithful to think He would reach out and catch you? No, that's called irresponsible. The book of Proverbs says: "The fear of the Lord is the beginning of knowledge and understanding." Without this basic understanding of your relationship and responsibility to the One who created you, life is just one health crisis after another.

The Bible is filled with leadership figures that were all blessed with the character of God through simple obedience. The will of God vs. the will of man, for most of us, is our greatest challenge. However, doing what we are *should do* versus what we *want to do* will always bring us freedom in the end. Thus, it has been said: "Discipline is Freedom."

While your past days may have been for better or worse, the good news is you get to start anew RIGHT NOW! Today is a new day that brings a new opportunity to be the best you can be. I find most folks encouraged by this simple, but powerful thought. So, let's get to it. First you need a plan. Not just any old plan, but a war plan to attack your new resolution full out- head on! My question to you is: If your plan last year wasn't so great, what will improve this year?

"The unexamined life is not worth living." – Plato

1. **Resolve to be more disciplined:** Commit to at least one healthy daily ritual, without wavering or missing it for anything or anyone. For you, this could mean exercise, eating a salad for lunch, or finding quiet time in your day consistently. Whatever it may be; *done* is better than perfect. Remember, faith is an act, and when you act CONSISTENTLY and in CONGRUENCY with your values, you build your character.

2. **Walk away from the 97% crowd. Don't use their excuses. Take charge of your own life:** If what they did worked, everyone's success in life and health would be the rule, not the exception. Unfortunately, today there's more financial and physical bankruptcy than ever. *"Be transformed by the renewing of your mind…"* Commit NOW to becoming a master at living a principled lifestyle: preceding every action with thought and alignment of God's laws of Love, Health, and Healing. This is THE ONLY WAY to achieve your true potential in life and health. I will personally teach you HOW in the following pages and at every monthly workshop event, leaving no stone unturned.

3. **Become a mentor:** Yes, YOU! Something powerful and amazing happens when you take on the responsibility of helping another; you inadvertently help yourself! Isolation and indifference is not only unhealthy, it leads to a life of mediocrity, depression, and despair. Helping your loved ones and friends find a new life in *"Elevation Health"* is an eternal gift that truly keeps on giving.

CHAPTER 2

Positive Programming

"Somehow I can't believe that there are any heights that can't be scaled by a man who knows the secrets of making dreams come true. This special secret - curiosity, confidence, courage, and constancy, and the greatest of all is confidence. When you believe in a thing, believe in it all the way, implicitly and unquestionable." — *Walt Disney*

There is no doubt that the one who believes the most achieves the most. In our quest for constant and never ending improvement, the ability to stay focused on the positive is the key to pushing us onward and upward. You see, the quality of our thoughts determine our emotions, our actions, and ultimately the results. Poor results lately? No miracle healings? Prayers seemingly remain unanswered? Check the "software" that you're choosing to run your mind with. I'll just use myself as an example: When I'm at my worst, I'm running the "Lack software". You know, the oh me, oh my story. "Oh, my back is killing me. Oh, I'm so tired. Oh, great- more bills!" And it just goes on and on without you even being aware that your language is actually creating your life conditions.

Conversely, when I'm at my absolute best all I'm thinking is ABUNDANCE, abundance, abundance, everywhere! If my back actually does hurt, what I've learned to do is speak words of gratitude *in advance* for the condition I see myself receiving. "I am grateful for a spine that is like a rod of iron. "Thank you for a back that is unbreakable and inexhaustible."

Life and Death is in the power of the tongue. The words you speak create the life you live, for better or worse. The major challenge here will be to unlearn the negative thought reactions associated with the different emotions we've been conditioned to cater to. When we exercise our freedom as intelligent human beings to *respond* rather than *react* to different emotions, we begin to choose LIFE. These are habits that may be hard to form. However, once in place, they are just as hard to break. The easiest way to do this is to create a ritual via your schedule. For example: After I wake up each day, my morning ritual is to read, pray, and exercise. This habit is as much a daily ritual as brushing my teeth. It happens the same time, each day, regardless of the day of the week. When I pray, my emotional state becomes that of GRATITUDE. This, I believe, is the key to living in abundance. When I exercise, I invigorate and energize my physical body, as well as sharpen my mental clarity. Good habits create outstanding character, which in turn breeds *leadership* for oneself- a necessary ingredient for success.

We are all creatures of habit, again, for better or worse. Bad habits create poor quality of life. Good habits create outstanding quality of life. I love the concept of know-ing that if I can be disciplined enough to do the things I'm supposed to do, then the success in my life is almost on autopilot. The word here is DISCIPLINE. This concept spans every aspect of blessing, joy, and wellbeing in our lives. Basically, we are all slaves to our habits. Why not be slave to the good habits that can unconsciously and effort-lessly lead us to obtaining our dreams?

James Allen wrote "Man becomes what he thinks about all day long." We need to own up to the mature understanding that WE are ultimately responsible for de-stroying our own lives with poorly chosen thoughts, words, and actions. The simple equation here: Poor choices = Poor results. Do you feel the negative vibration of your emotions as you read this sentence? For me, it stirs up a feeling of dissatisfaction, something that needs "a little fixin'." If it does for you as well, then we're on the right track. People are either motivated by one of two things: Pain or Pleasure. If things in your life need a little fixin' these days, then you're probably feeling the pain now of some poor choices or lack of discipline from the past. I want you to know this is a great starting point. Personally, I do well when realizing a certain sense of dissatisfaction in an area of my life. It gets me rallied up to the challenge of applying a new skill or mindset as a catalyst for change. I dislike change just as much as the next person. However, I've conditioned my mind to understand that not only is change inevitable, it's necessary for continued growth and personal achievement. Remember, healthy thoughts-healthy results.

The flip side of the coin for motivation we said was pleasure. The great news here is that nothing attracts success like success. When good things begin to happen over and over in your life, you realize at some point it's not by accident. You have now cracked the code for success; Doing what you are supposed to do when you are supposed to do it, to have what you want to have when you want to have it! We have now come full circle in the cycle of success: 1) Positive Belief in your Vision 2) Positive Thoughts. 3) Positive Language and Actions. 4) Positive Results.

CHAPTER 3

Planning For Success

"All great successes are the triumph of persistence."
— Ralph Waldow Emerson

A college professor once told me: "If you fail to plan, you plan to fail." It didn't take much brainpower to instantly realize the brilliance of this mindset. While I applied this concept to budgeting my time to prepare for exams, I also began to use it in all areas of life. I saw that most people are too busy drowning in the minutia of the day, to take time to plan and design the outcome in life they would like.

Every 12 weeks or so, I'd hop in my little Honda and drive from Atlanta to Miami to visit family. During these 11 hour trips the time would speed by as I reminisced about the past as well as thought about my future. I remember very vividly visualizing what my life would be like in 10 or 20 years; what my family would look like, how many kids I'd have, what type and size of practice I'd be in, financial goals, etc. The overwhelming emotions of encouragement, empowerment, and anticipation this exercise provided me with was powerful enough to propel me from where I was in life to where I wanted to be. I believed so strongly in my ability to achieve any level of success, so long as I maintained the discipline to focus, as well as scheduling the time to prepare. From then on, I always had my life plan in writing.

Whether, it's taking and exam, getting a college degree, starting a new job or even your own business; we all possess the same potential for success. The difference between success and failure begins between the ears, goes into the schedule, and finally ends with massive action. We can dream all day long, but without action, that dream often dies on the vine. Walt Disney took his vision and dreams to the pen and paper. When this happens, it's no longer exists as a dream, but a rather a seedling of reality. This is an astonishing fact if you think about all of the most amazing dreams and wishes you have for your life. How many of them could possibly begin to exist if you were to write them out as goals? If you could see these goals in written form, isn't it possible that you could write out a few action steps that would move you toward achieving these goals? I say this because most of our brains today are in overload from the daily bombardment of little useless details. Memory management usually fails us. Thus, when it comes to "planning for success", Rule #1 is: Your goals and dreams must be IN WRITING. Bottom line is, if it's not written, then it's not real.

These days, regular planning is programmed into my daily, weekly, monthly, and yearly calendar. Usually around October, I begin to plan out the following year, both personally and professionally. Top values such as family vacations, seminars and coaching, and finally our monthly office Power Workshops go first. Any other monthly events may then go around that. Weekly planning happens on Sunday morning. As I scan the meetings and events on my calendar for that week, I dial in the tasks that need to be executed on the appropriate day necessary for optimal outcome. The stress of last minute details is minimized utilizing this discipline. Thus, on any given weekday, I have a task list on my daily planner reminding me of what needs to be done and why I need to do it.

They say success is in the details. I cannot over emphasize this statement. For some it may be too much. However, no one ever told me success comes easy. The extra discipline and effort here, over time, simply becomes a habit that unconsciously carries you to the place of your dreams. Success in life doesn't happen by hopes or chance, it is something that must be PLANNED. If your life is worth living, then it's worth planning.

Top 3 Joy Stealers

1. Focusing on what you can't control or influence: ie) traffic, weather, past, people's words and deeds.
2. News and World Events, Emotional Challenges, Treatment for Illness
3. Lack of Planning, Organizing, Coaching and Maintenance

Discipline is the Bridge between Inspiration and Achievement. Discipline comes from the root word *Disciple*. In the Bible the "Disciples" were noted for not necessarily doing what they wanted to do, but rather WHAT THEY *HAD TO DO* FOR GOD. This is the single handed explanation for the Gospel reaching around the Globe starting with only 12 people.

Commitment leads not to sacrifice, but a life filled with Joy. Being committed to a cause *greater than yourself* releases the Power of Joy in your life greater than can be imagined. Simply put: The Servant's Life is a Life of Joy. The bible says "to be greatest among all is to be servant of all"; your family, co-workers, and friends, etc. This life leaves no room to be stressed- only BLESSED!

The Solution: scheduling more consistent time for:
   1) Faith
   2) Family/ Relationship Building
   3) Fitness/Healthy Lifestyle: proper nutrition, exercise, and regular family wellness checkups.
   4) Finances

   Creating and sustaining the character habits of discipline, commitment, and obedience in all areas of your life will create an outstanding life of joy, health and prosperity- leaving little room for stress.

CHAPTER 4

Mission Mindedness

"Man's greatness is measured by what you see in others and how you bring it out of them." — unknown

In the movie "World Trade Center", Nicolas cage and Michael Pena play two New York City policemen trapped under 25 feet of massive rubble on September 11, 2001. With concrete crushing them, and explosions all around, they fight for their lives wounded and dehydrated. Finally, the search and rescue team locates them. A Marine is at the top of the rubble calling down to one of them. One officer begs, "Please don't leave us, we've been here for days." To which his response was, "It's O.K., I'm a Marine. You ARE MY MISSION."

That was a WOW moment for me. I really connected with that sort of purpose in my life. Day in and day out I pray that God would send me the sick and suffering; those hurting and in need of healing. In our office, we see people coming from different cities, states, and sometimes different countries to receive the unique gift of healing and compassion my team and I have been blessed with. Why? Because there's never been a greater need in the history of mankind. There is, without a doubt, more sickness and disease devastating our families than ever before.

Each week I speak in the community at a different place of work or worship. Why? Because THE PEOPLE ARE MY MISSION. With as much high blood pressure, cholesterol, diabetes, and depression as there is right now, I'm not OK with just sitting in my office, hoping these people live long enough to get my help. My community workshops are *search and rescue missions* for the millions of people that will die a miserable early death if I don't get to them in time. Most of these people have been living on the medical merry-go-round; going from one doctor to the next, from one drug to the next, continuing to develop more and more disease. To me, they are all "trapped under the rubble", and praying for a way out.

At each event, I always have people approach me looking for solutions to their health challenges. There exists a major lack for knowledge in the realm of health and healing today. Day after day, I hear the cries of the people: "My doctor gave me a prescription for Lipitor, and I really hate taking drugs. Is there anything else that will help me?" "My husband was just admitted to the hospital for diabetes. The doctors said he'll need to be on meds for the rest of his life." "My mother has just been diagnosed with breast cancer, and we don't want to do the chemotherapy; is there anything else?"

To me, they are all the same questions with the same answer: YES! YES! YES! There is another way. And all it requires is obtaining a little wisdom and knowledge, and then applying it. In Proverbs 3:13-14, Solomon claims this to be of better profit than silver or gold. Of course! People would pay anything to have their health back once they lose it. Unfortunately, oftentimes, people wait until it's too late. My responsibility, as I see it, is to make sure that every man, woman, and child in my town has heard the story about Health and Healing and moreover been given the opportunity to live a long life of abundant health and vitality.

As a result of being *Mission Minded*, we have been blessed with one of the largest natural healing facilities in the world. We have a very busy office, and we like it that way. The busier we are, the more lives we know are being saved. It is as simple as that.

When you finally take your eyes off of you, and begin to focus on serving and loving your neighbor, therein lies your treasure. You forget about your woes, and get lost in the blessings and joy that are created in the moments of pure unadulterated, selfless service. If you've never felt that, you should try it sometime. Volunteer at a soup kitchen, a homeless shelter, your temple or church outreach ministry, or even just to share with someone how much they mean to you. These are all acts of service and compassion, and when acted upon, we become instruments for God's purpose and plan for humankind.

For purposes of this book, having a servant's heart is really the key to unlocking the vault to overwhelming success and joy in all areas of one's life. Whatever your career, business, or mission in life may be, it is impossible to fail if your primary purpose is to serve. If helping people get what they want is your mission, then finding more ways to serve more people becomes the only limit to your success.

CHAPTER **5**

Letting Go Of Fear

"Faith is the hostess that will not entertain doubt."
— Jenna Wright

There isn't one person alive who hasn't experienced the taste of fear. If you're like me, fear is probably a regular guest in your life. However, I am aware of the fact that I possess the power to choose whether or not I will host such a guest in my life or dismiss it. A spirit of excellence and mastery will quickly discern fear as a breakthrough opportunity to massive growth in one's life. Tragically, most never acquire the wisdom to identify this opportunity. You see, Fear comes to us in disguise. Wearing the battle scars, woes, and defeat of those who've seemingly failed before us, fear sounds most like the voice of reason. However, this impostor is not to be confused with the voice of reason and truth. You must be strong in your daily walk to discern the difference.

With the right perspective, you can turn your fear into

fuel; the greater the fear, the greater the fuel to propel you to your destiny; the greater the fear, the greater the courage that is needed to overcome it. Courage is the character of God. In the Old Testament, Joshua 1:9 says: "Have I not commanded thee? Be strong and of good courage; be not afraid, neither be thou dismayed: for the Lord thy God is with thee withersoever thou goest." The Promised Land being a land filled with giants, I'm sure was reason enough for Joshua to be fearful. However, the Lord spoke to him and gave him courage. When we have the courage to do something that is uncomfortable or fearful, we are allowing God to build His character within us. This is the key to opening the door for the greatest blessings in life.

Several years ago, I was in practice with a partner. We had a built a very successful practice together, running strong for about 7 years. Things were seemingly going well on the surface, but something was not right in my heart. I began to search for the reason why I was feeling this way, and I kept coming up with the same answer: "Time to spread your wings and fly," was the call in my heart. But the "voice of reason" kept telling me it didn't make sense, as I had a good practice going, making a good living, nice house, nice car, newly married with a baby, etc... Why would I put all of that at risk when things were "good enough" as they were? I didn't have all the answers, so I began to pray. My wife, Yvette, and I would sit in bed at night and talk it through. I remember my exact words to her expressing my fear about the situation: I said, "Honey, I feel like I'm standing on the edge of a cliff looking down, and there's no turning back. I have to launch out now, and I'm either going down hard, or God is going to be the wind beneath my wings taking me to new heights."

The rest is history. Within 2 weeks I had located another office space to practice in. A moving chiropractor basically gave me his office already built out. Within 2 months, we made the physical move to the new address seeing 250 patients per week. Within 6 months, the practice swelled to over 650 patients per week, and continued to climb to over 1100 patients per week. While the average clinic sees about 100 per week, God had blessed me tenfold for my courage and obedience. Sometimes you receive such a blessing that it's humbling and overwhelming all at the same time. It took me some time to get comfortable with this new level of responsibility and leadership. However, I soon realized that it was all part of being led to my destiny. The courage that was required to conquer my fear is the same courage required to create strong leadership. This is exactly my calling in life: I am a leader for my community- to help the sick get well, and the well to stay healthy. I am a leader for my family, for my staff, and for all around me that need leadership, positive influence, and stability. I realize that I am far from perfect, however, as a leader I choose to be disciplined and obedient to the call of God's will in my life, and the daily preparations necessary to achieve it.

Beware the voice of "good enough", as it comes as a thief in the night to rob us of our destiny. Good enough usually means its good enough *for you*. That's fine if your only purpose in life is to serve yourself. However, if your purpose in life is to serve a Higher Call, then good enough seldom is. A true servant- leader is never done serving, as his heart is always looking to help others. Maintaining a fearless and courageous character will always prepare you for greater opportunities- greater than the mind can conceive.

<u>NEVER, EVER, EVER, EVER, EVER GIVE UP!</u>

"When things go wrong as they sometimes will,
When the road you're trudging seems all uphill.
When the funds are low and the debts are high,
And you want to smile but you have to sigh.
When care is pressing you down a bit,
Rest if you must, but don't you quit.

Life is queer with its twists and turns,
As every one of us sometimes learns.
And many a fellow turns about,
When he might have won had he stuck it out.
Don't give up though the pace seems slow,
You may succeed with another blow.

Often the goal is nearer than
It seems to a faint and faltering man.
Often the struggler has given up,
When he might have captured the victor's cup.
And he learned too late when the night came down,
How close he was to the golden crown.

Success is failure turned inside out,
The silver tint of the clouds of doubt.
And you never can tell how close you are,
It may be near when it seems afar.
So stick to the fight when you're hardest hit,
It's when things seem worst that you mustn't quit.
...And that's worth thinking about!"

Part Two

Energizing Nutrition

Strengthening the Inner Foundation

CHAPTER 1

Balancing the Blood

If I could live my life over again, I would devote it to proving that germs seek their natural habitat- diseased tissue- rather than being the cause of diseased tissue; e.g., mosquitoes seek the stagnant water, but do not cause the pool to become stagnant.
— Rudolph Virchow (Father of Pathology)

Imagine a river flowing through a beautiful countryside where a growing community thrives. That river is a lifeline for people providing a source of water, food, bathing, and a myriad of other life- sustaining necessities. Unless, of course, toxins or poisons are introduced into the streaming water, then we have major problem. If the river becomes toxic, what was once a wellspring for life now becomes a source for sickness, disease, and death.

The same can be said of the human bloodstream; under healthy conditions, it is a life- sustaining river bringing a steady flow of fresh oxygen, nutrients, and disease fighting agents to all vital tissues and organs of the body. That is, until the blood becomes toxic; then we have the beginning of a serious problem. What was intended to be the wellspring for outrageous health, increasing energy, and amazing vitality, now becomes a toxic dump- a fertile breeding ground for bacteria, viruses, fungus, yeast, and mold to thrive in. In essence, they are living off of dying, decaying matter. These living agents continue to thrive, excrete more toxins in the bloodstream, and aid in perpetuating a downward spiral of degenerative disease in the body.

Toxicity of the bloodstream can lead to the exhibition of virtually any symptom or disease known to mankind. Headaches, nausea, dizziness, fatigue, depression, difficulty breathing, fibromyalgia, and chronic aches and pains of the back and joints are some of the most common signs of blood toxicity. Over long periods of time, it may also lead to clogging of the arteries, high blood pressure, high cholesterol, diabetes, obesity, and cancer.

Maintaining proper blood pH is essential for optimal health. Normal blood ph is slightly alkaline- 7.365. Some acidic conditions in the body are necessary such as digestion and kidney function. Outside of this, however, most lifestyles today contribute to an acidic blood pH, which creates a perfect environment to sustain life for bacteria, viruses, yeast, mold, and fungus. It is this acidic environment that also plays host to so many diseases that we suffer from today. Cancer, arteriosclerosis, high blood pressure, high cholesterol, depression, chronic fatigue, obesity all result from living an acid diet and lifestyle.

Typical alkaline foods are lettuce, broccoli, cauliflower, spinach, celery, cucumbers, garlic, cabbage, peas, onions, asparagus, sprouts and greens of all kinds. Generally speaking, the greener they are, the better they are for you. Other alkaline foods would be Omega 3 oils such as flax oil, fish oils, extra virgin olive oil, and cod liver oil. Additionally, certain bottled waters may fall into the alkalizing category as well.

On the other end of the pH scale, we have all the foods that contribute to acidification of the body. Some of these typically include all sugars, salt, vinegar, alcohol, nicotine, dairy, meat, refined and/ or flour enriched products (white pasta, white rice, white bread), and prescription/ over the counter medication.

As you may be wondering if it is possible to avoid all of these foods, stop and realize that this is not going to happen overnight. For most folks, the process of learning and applying new knowledge takes time; it must be an evolution- a gradual change in lifestyle. First we start with the knowledge.

I have been witness to so many of our patients watch their blood pressure drop 40 points, their blood sugar drop 100 points, and cholesterol come down over 100 points when these principles are applied with discipline.

Live blood cell microscopy has demonstrated the effect of acid conditions in the bloodstream – in particular, the effect on blood cells. For example, red blood cells have a bi-lipid layer of fat making up the cell wall. The inside of the cell is positively charged, while the outside of the cell wall bears a negative charge. The external cell wall nega-tive charge serves the purpose of repelling each red blood cell from another so that they travel at maximum velocity through the blood vessel and may enter single file in to the capillaries and tissues. This scenario occurs under normal blood pH conditions, thereby delivering maximum oxygen to the tissues, resulting in maximum energy, vitality, resistance to disease, and healing.

A converse situation exists with an acidic bloodstream: Let's take for example a can of soft drink which typically contains sugar, high fructose corn syrup, and caffeine (the perfect acid cocktail). The sugar ingested, digested, and sent to the blood stream has broken down directly into acid. The intensive acid medium in the bloodstream now begins to erode and breakdown the cell walls. As these cell walls are merely made of fat, the emulsification process takes little time before the integrity of the cell wall is completely destroyed and all of the positive charges contained within the cell are released. As this occurs, the polarity of the outer cell wall now becomes reversed, creating a positive charge around all of the red blood cells. As a result, the cells are now attracted to one another, clumping together, now moving ever so slowly through the bloodstream. The result is less oxygenation to the tissues, leading to less energy, foggy thinking, less vitality, lowered resistance to disease and infection, and an overall decrease in healing ability.

I usually use a power point animation to illustrate these effects while lecturing to groups. Everyone is always amazed at how much this makes sense. But what really blows people away is when we further illustrate what the blood vessels begin to look like with all of these blood cells clumping and sticking together over long periods of time. After decades of accumulation of damaged blood cells sticking together, they have long been sticking to the artery walls. This type of artery clogging, or plaque may lead to high blood pressure and/ or stroke.

Remember we mentioned that the cell walls that are made of fat are destroyed by the acid environment. Because we were created with an Innate Intelligence, the body goes to work repairing the cell walls by producing more cholesterol. As a means of healing and protection, cholesterol is a necessary part of everyone's normal body chemistry. It just make sense that the overly acidic person will have much higher blood cholesterol levels as the body attempts to survive under toxic conditions.

Along the same lines, an acid diet and lifestyle is linked to weight gain and obesity. Regardless of all the fat you may cut out of your diet to lose weight, your body will not let go of that excess fat because it needs it to rebuild, repair, and protect the damaged cells from acidity and toxicity.

CHAPTER **2**

Alkalizing and Energizing

"The important thing is this: To be able at any moment to sacrifice what we are for what we could become."
— Charles du Bois

One of THE most valuable commodities an individual may possess is energy. Think for a moment what happens when you have more energy; you feel better, you think more clearly, you make better decisions, you're more productive, more profitable, your value increases exponentially in the marketplace, as a parent, and as a contributor to society, in general. With productivity comes an increase in character, in turn generating increase in fulfillment, resulting in more joy.

Energy is the necessary fuel to reach any level of success and fulfillment in anyone's life. Be assured that NASCAR drivers do not take their cars to the track on race day, fill it up with regular gasoline, and expect to win the race. High performance vehicles demand high octane fuels which merely enable them to compete, much less win a race.

In the same way, most of us lead high performance lives with demanding jobs, demanding kids, demanding spouses, demanding homes with high maintenance. If we are ever to keep up with the race of life, then we need the right fuels. If you want to compete at a high level, and determined to succeed, you need high octane fuels to run the body.

The choices that we make regarding what enters our body, will single-handedly determine the outcome of your day, week, month, year, and overall life. Your wealth, health, and longevity hinge on the actions you take from nutritional breakthroughs, such as contained in this book. Choosing the right foods to promote the right blood pH will yield an immediate increase in your energy, vitality, and overall sense of well being. It happens that fast!

When out in the community putting on these workshops, I often emphasize that Rome was not build in a day; therefore don't expect your diet to change radically overnight. However, if we can add just a few good things to your diet, you'll begin to see great changes instantly.

MORE GREENS:

Most of us can still remember the food pyramid we learned in elementary school. The bottom of the pyramid represented 60% of foods consumed in our daily diet. Do you remember what that was? That's right- carbohydrates: Breads, pastas, cereals, and grains. That single recommendation is responsible for 1 million new cases of diabetes each year. Right now 60 million Americans are either diabetic or pre-diabetic. More people are on more diabetes drugs than ever. Why? Lifestyle; Eating too much and eating too much of the wrong carbohydrates. Medical studies now show that diabetics have the highest risk of Alzheimer's disease. Eating a diet high in refined carbohydrates significantly increases ones risk of pre-cognitive decline, dementia, and Alzheimer's disease.

Ideally, our diet should be made up of at least 60% greens. This is what needs to be changed and taught in our schools. What makes greens the color green is the chlorophyll these foods contain. Through a process known as photosynthesis plants convert light into energy. The conversion of unusable sunlight energy into usable chemical energy is associated with the actions of the green pigment chlorophyll. Thus, the simplicity of the dietary equation; More greens = More energy. Additionally, most greens and green vegetables break down to an alkaline ash in the bloodstream. This helps to maintain the proper blood pH necessary for maintaining health and resisting disease.

A typical daily diet example for me would look like the following: Upon waking, an 8 oz cup of coffee and then workout. 40 minutes later I'll have a protein shake with coconut milk, 2 scoops of almond butter and some berries. At 10 am I have a Granny Smith apple. For lunch I'll have a large mixed green salad with olive oil and pink salt, and a scoop of tuna fish or chicken salad on top. At 3:30, I'll have vegan protein shake with a handful of almonds. At around 6:30, we have dinner which is always just meat and vegetables. Last night we had baked chicken breasts and green beans with peas. On all vegetables, I always use a generous serving of extra virgin olive oil or organic butter with a sprinkle of pink salt. Other week nights, I usually enjoy a variety of fresh fish and vegetables. Salmon, Cod, Grouper, and Sea Bass are my preference. However, there are plenty of omega-3 rich fish to choose from; Tuna, Halibut, and Sardines fit the bill, as well. With my meat portions, I'll frequently have some sort of starchy vegetable carbohydrate such as peas, squash, broccoli, cauliflower, or sweet potato. Again, with all vegetable servings, for my entire family; we always top them off with the lots of real organic butter or extra virgin olive oil. This balances the meal with the necessary essential fats, aids in digestion, promotes more stable blood sugar levels, promotes healthy new cells, aids in proper brain function, and balances blood pressure and cholesterol, not to mention tastes great!

I recommend not drinking liquids with meals so as to avoid disrupting normal digestion. Post meal beverages (slightly acidic) may be enjoyed to aid with digestion as well. This would include tea, organic coffee, or apple cider vinegar.

MORE FAT:

The right amount of the right fat will not only serve to repair and protect the red blood cells and tissues, it will also help your body release unwanted excess fat as well. Recall that the cell walls are made up of fat. As the acid breaks down those cell walls, the body creates more fat (cholesterol) and maintains excess body fat for utilization in the cellular repair and regeneration process. Simply put: if you want to lose fat, you must eat fat! Good fat, that is. Of course, man made trans fats in French fries, potato chips, and baked goods do not qualify for this category. The right fats we are speaking of are Omega rich essential fats. This would include healthy monounsaturated oils such as extra virgin olive oil, cold pressed flax seed oil, fish oils, and cod liver oil just to name a few. Foods rich in these oils range from almonds and avocados to fresh fish such as salmon, cod, tuna, halibut, and sardines, in addition to real butter, and grass fed meats. Recent studies continue to prove these healthy fats benefit the body in a myriad of other ways including:

- Aids in digestion
- Stabilizes blood sugar
- Lowers blood pressure
- Lowers cholesterol & triglycerides
- Prevents cancer
- Natural anti-inflammatory
- Improves brain function
- Helps fight depression
- Promotes healthy skin

As far as "bang for the buck", few supplements even come close to all of the life- saving, disease- preventing benefits of these oils if taken 2-3 times daily as a liquid or capsule dietary supplement. Personally, my daily routing consists of 2 fish oil capsules at lunch time, sometimes a tablespoon of coconut oil or butter in my coffee, and of course generous servings of extra virgin olive oil on greens at meals.

If you are still wondering about the coconut oil; this is a medium chain triglyceride which the body actually processes like sugar. This provides sustainable energy as well as powerful fat- burning benefits.

This is one of the best kept fat burning secrets!

Equally as important, it should be noted that these

good fats provide the body with incredible amounts of pure sustainable quantities of energy. As opposed to the quick burning bursts of energy that sugar provides, fat, on the other hand has a slow burning mechanism for providing its energy. When I was training for the Disney Marathon several years ago, my coach at the time, Stu Mittleman, shared with me a vivid analogy; He said that the energy we get from sugar is like the phosphates of a matchstick-lighting up and burning out quickly. However, the energy we get from fat is like the coals on a barbeque- slow to get burning, but nearly impossible to put out! This proved to be more than accurate relative to his advice with preparation for the day of the 26.2 mile race. While 20,000 other runners were out the night before carb loading pasta and pancakes, I was eating salmon and jasmine rice, with a large serving of vegetables loaded with extra virgin olive oil. On race day, I was nibbling on water soaked almonds during the entire 5 hour race. Ultimately, Stu's wisdom proved superior to conventional, as I finished the race strong and injury free. Moreover, while most marathoners finish a race and spend the next week recuperating with daily massages, hot tub treatments, and bed rest, I was back to work the next day with flying colors; I never missed a beat! The power of good fats in your diet cannot be overstated.

MORE WATER:

Most of us have been told that 8 glasses a day will keep the doctor away. Unfortunately, due to today's extremely acidic diet and lifestyle, this amount tends to fall short. Additionally, for most folks, many of those 8 glasses tend to get substituted for tea, juice, soda, and coffee. The correct amount of daily water consumption, in general, should be half of your body weight in fluid ounces. This would mean that a 200 lb individual should drink approximately 100oz. per day. This would equate to roughly 3 liters.

For eons, water has been used and touted as a multicure, natural wonder. This makes sense, due to the fact that dehydration can cause cellular dysfunction of any or all tissues and organs in the body. Lack of water in the bloodstream causes a lack of protection for the cells from the damaging effects of acid breakdown. In much the same way fat protects ands creates a buffer for cellular repair and regeneration, so it is true of water. This makes drinking water, for most people with health challenges, such a no brainer. It's cheap, easy, and user- friendly, with zero side- effects!

CHAPTER 3

Food By Man

"If I knew I was going to live this long, I'd have taken better care of myself."
— Mickey Mantle

For most of us, our meals of the day consist of self- indulging events that look and taste great but leave us feeling guilty and lethargic in less than one hour flat. Immediate gratification has and always will be the weak link for humankind in multiple areas of life, particularly relative to one's health. Funny, though, how quickly everyone will agree that delayed gratification always yields sweeter and greater long term rewards.

As we've learned up to this point, there are certain foods that work well with the body, and certain foods that don't. The issues of health and longevity can be solved by learning the difference between the two, and having the discipline to choose wisely.

A simple rule of thumb I always teach is "if man made

it, don't eat it." Real foods are perfect unto themselves packed with vitamins, minerals, and antioxidants essential for the maintenance of human health and life. We know these foods all too well; all the fruits and veggies that we've been taught about since childhood, but never quite get enough of: Cauliflower, Broccoli, Peas, Carrots, Squash, Brussels Sprouts, Tomatoes, Lettuce, Cucumbers, and Spinach are some of the more common and traditional vegetables that come to mind. Fruits, of course, have always enjoyed more fanfare. Apples, oranges, bananas, melons, and berries, not only taste great, but are amazingly healthy. What do these fruits and vegetables have in common? They typically can be harvested from the soil or picked from the vine and ready to eat without anything man-made to add to it.

In contrast man made foods are not naturally grown or harvested, and therefore require additives for taste, preservatives for shelf life, colorings for aesthetics, and artificial ingredients to make them biologically consumable. The problem is, what is not natural truly does not belong in the body. In other words, if God didn't make it, then don't eat it. Ignoring this rule of thumb has painful health consequences.

Preservatives in our foods do not allow your body to digest that food. Hydrogenated oils and fats are well known to cause heart disease, and in fact, now have their own death category. Perfect examples of these are Twinkie's or fast food hamburgers after one year sitting on a shelf in your garage. There's no mold or decay. These synthetic fats are like synthetic oils; they never break down. MSG is a neurotoxin hidden in most foods to create addiction to the product. It has long been known to cause hypertension, in addition to other organ dysfunction. These, among other unnatural added ingredients in our foods today, all cause immediate damage in the body.

Typical man made foods are all the ones we've come to know and love such as white bread, white rice, and white pasta. All of these foods pass through a bleaching and refinement process that strips away nearly all of the vitamins, nutrients and minerals. In addition, such starchy carbohydrates break down into sugar that causes insulin levels to skyrocket. Increased insulin levels is not only associated with diabetes, but with increased body fat, weight loss resistance, and overall fatigue. When the hormone insulin increases as a result of these sugars, a destructive metabolic process is now under way. Your body now begins assembling triglycerides (fat) in the bloodstream contributing to the process of heart attack and stroke. Powerful inflammatory compounds known as cytokines are released causing artery walls to swell which increases blood pressure. Lastly, when insulin is elevated, another hormone called Leptin is raised further contributing to weight loss resistance.

Dairy...what the dairy industry never told you

One of the greatest hoaxes ever perpetuated upon mankind is that of the dairy industry. Through generations of clever marketing and advertising, it is now a common belief that dairy is an absolute part of our diets, for children and adults. Rarely does a mother pass by the supermarket dairy section without feeling good about bringing home a few gallons of milk and cheese to keep the family healthy.

Why? Because everyone knows that you need Vitamin D and Calcium for strong healthy bones and teeth. And where have we been taught that comes from? That's right, milk.

Think about this, though, for just a moment. The United States consumes more milk each year than any other country in the world, yet we boast the highest rate of osteoporosis diagnosed each year! I believe there are two reasons for this: 1) The typical American diet is void of the optimal amount of daily greens consumed, which is naturally rich with all the calcium one would ever need for strong, healthy bones and teeth. 2) Commercially produced milk is loaded with the sugar Lactose, the breakdown of which results in acidification of the bloodstream and blood cells. The condition of over-acidification in the bloodstream causes leeching of calcium from the bones which leads to osteoporosis.

Additionally, commercial dairy is high in omega-6 essential fatty acids which have long been associated with inflammation of the mucosal membranes. Most particularly affected by this are the nasal and sinus cavities; resulting in inflammation of the sinuses, sinus infections, asthma, and allergies. Fully, 60% of all patients walking into my office have these symptoms, most of which have their cause from a diet high in dairy. It's amazing how apparent this is when I address the nutritional habits of parents concerning their children. We always find that when removing the dietary dairy, the results for improved breathing are significant in nearly all cases. In most cases it's quite apparent; a bowl of cereal with milk everyday for breakfast, a cheese pizza, an omelet with cheese, lunch meats with cheese, grated or shredded cheeses on salads and dinners. The long list of lurking causes usually continues unexamined.

Another issue not to be overlooked is how modern day livestock are fed. Grain fed cattle and poultry make for larger, healthier, and more valuable livestock, however, the price humans pay at the other end of the food chain is dearly regrettable. Along with all of the grain these animals ingest come a long list of powerful biotoxins in the form of pesticides, herbicides, steroids, hormones and antibiotics. This inherently becomes part of the food we eat and ultimately translates to sickness, disease, and dysfunction on a cellular level.

This however, does not mean that I recommend avoiding all meats and dairy. I do recommend, rather organic grass fed meats and dairy products in moderation as part of a well balanced diet. Organic, grass fed meat and dairy is by far the healthier choice, as you get to by-pass the harmful effects of biotoxins, and you actually get to enjoy the proper Omega- 3 fatty ratios of 4:1 helping to stave off many of the deadly degenerative diseases we suffer from today.

More on Grain Fed vs. Grass Fed Meat

When animals eat grain it changes the very important fat ratio in the meat. A North Dakota State University study determined that the omega 6 to omega 3 ratios is 4 to 1 in **grass-fed** animals. This important ratio was determined to be 21 to 1 in **grain-fed** animals. The World Health Organization has determined that the 4 to 1 Omega 6 to Omega 3 ratio is the optimal ratio at the cellular level.

In the 2003 Yehuda study, participants who were treated with proper Omega fatty ratios experienced:

- Decreased M.S. symptoms.
- Improved sleep quality.
- Decreased ADD and ADHD symptoms.
- Increase stress adaptation by decreasing Cortisol levels.
- Improved cognitive function thus learning ability.

No other fatty acid ratio produced the above benefits.

An additional concern to be noted is what has been referred to as the **law of biological concentration**. That is; it takes about 5 to 8 pounds of chemically sprayed grain to produce 1 pound of beef. Thus, you will ingest considerably *more cancer causing chemicals from meat* than from fruit and vegetables.

One of the most impactful changes you can make that will immediately impact your overall health and well being is to start consuming grass fed meat (buffalo, elk, veal). This will have a significant anti- inflammatory effect at the cellular level to allow for healing of nearly all lifestyle re-lated degenerative diseases such as: High blood pressure, high cholesterol, diabetes, obesity, insomnia, and brain/learning disorders.

Fat and Disease

All studies that have linked fat to disease never differ-entiated between good fat and bad fat. The following may be classified as the Bad fats:

- Hydrogenated and Partially Hydrogenated Oils: *cottonseed oil, soybean oil, vegetable oils.*
- Trans Fats: *margarine and synthetic butters.*

- Rancid Vegetable Oils: *"corn oil"*, *canola oil, or those labeled simply vegetable oil. Found in practically every bread, cracker, cookie, and boxed food.*
- Fats in Grain- Fed Meat:

Bad fats eventually lead to the causation of:
1. Cellular Congestion – leading to cellular dysfunction and therefore cancer.
2. Inflammation of the Arteries – heart attacks and stroke.
3. Decrease in Nerve Function –decrease in focus, increase in hyperactivity and depression.

CHAPTER 4

Toxins By Man

"Victory belongs to the most persevering."
— Napoleon Bonaparte

Cholesterol Drugs: Curing or Causing Disease?

The Dangers of Cholesterol Lowering Drugs:

1- The journal **Nature Medicine** found that statin drugs produced significant depression of T- helper cells (white blood cells). These cells play a vital role in protection from cancer, viral, bacterial, and fungal infections. This puts an individual at higher risk for developing infections. Additionally, chronic immune suppression puts an individual at significantly higher risk for developing cancer, and those already with cancer would see tremendous growth and spread of their cancers. *All statin drugs have been associated with causing and promoting cancer in experimental animals.*

2 - **The heart muscle** is extremely dependent on the energy molecule CoQ10. All statin drugs dramatically lower CoQ10 levels. <u>Since the introduction of these drugs, there has been a 600% increase in congestive heart failure.</u>

3- **The American Heart Association** found that people taking statin cholesterol lowering drugs had increased difficulty performing everyday tasks such as driving a car. These individuals were found to have attention problems, delayed reflexes, difficulty thinking, and memory loss. Researchers found that the lower the cholesterol, the worse the effects.

4- **For years the recommended blood cholesterol was in the range of 200- 210 mg/dl.** Why the recent change? Simple: At nearly 70 million Americans on these drugs, just do the math. Cholesterol drugs alone gross more than $20 billion a year for the drug companies.

If you or anyone you know are taking any of these common cholesterol lowering drugs such as Liptor, Mevacor, Prevachol, or Zocor, ask your doctor why they have not yet brought this information to your attention. Then ask them: considering the devastating side effects, and the fact that *it doesn't correct the cause of the problem*, how long they intend to keep you on these drugs. Finally, the golden question: If it's not correcting the cause, then what are you doing to really help me?

The Only True Cure: *Correcting the Cause*

1. **Proper nerve supply** to your liver and all other organs ensures that your body makes the right amount of cholesterol for YOU- *no more and no less.*

2. **Proper Nutrition and Supplementation:** A **daily** multivitamin, **CoQ10** (150 mg/day), **Vit. C** (1000mg, 3/day), **Vit. D3** (1000 IU/day), **Green Tea extract**, and Grape Seed extract (100mg/day each), **L- Carnitine** (500 mg/day on empty stomach). Additionally, eating a healthy **Alkaline diet** will not only reduce your risk of heart disease, but cancer, diabetes, depression, and obesity as well.

3. **Daily Exercise:** Brisk walking with resistance training on alternating days has proven to be of greatest physiological benefit overall for maximizing health and minimizing the risk of degenerative disease. 20- 30 min. is recommended.

The Benefits of High Cholesterol

People with high cholesterol live the longest: Consider the finding of Dr. Harlan Krumholz of the Department of Cardiovascular Medicine at Yale University, who reported in 1994 that old people **with low cholesterol died twice as often from a heart attack as did old people with a high cholesterol.**[1]

Most studies of old people have shown that **high**

---

1   Krumholz HM and others. Lack of association between cholesterol and coronary heart disease mortality and morbidity and all-cause mortality in persons older than 70 years. *Journal of the American Medical Association* 272, 1335-1340, 1990.

cholesterol is not a risk factor for coronary heart disease. Eleven studies of old people came up with that result, and a further seven studies found that high cholesterol did not predict all-cause mortality either.

High Cholesterol Protects against Infection: Many studies have found that low cholesterol is in certain respects worse than high cholesterol. For instance, in 19 large studies of more than 68,000 deaths, reviewed by Professor David R. Jacobs and his co-workers from the Division of Epidemiology at the University of Minnesota, **low cholesterol predicted an increased risk of dying from gastrointestinal and respiratory diseases**. Ravnskov U. High cholesterol may protect against infections and atherosclerosis. *Quarterly Journal of Medicine* 96, 927-934, 2003.

Low Cholesterol and HIV/AIDS: Results come from a study of more than 300,000 young and middle-aged men, which found that the number of men (whose cholesterol was lower than 160 and who had died from AIDS) was four times higher than the number of men who had died from AIDS with a cholesterol above 240.7 Claxton AJ and others. Association between serum total cholesterol and HIV infection in a high-risk cohort of young men. *Journal of acquired immune deficiency syndromes and human retrovirology* 17, 51–57, 1998.

Cholesterol and Chronic Heart Failure: The largest study has been performed by Professor Gregg C. Fonorow and his team at the UCLA Department of Medicine and Cardiomyopathy Center in Los Angeles.[13] The study, led by Dr. Tamara Horwich, included more than a thousand patients with severe heart failure. <u>After five years 62 percent of the patients with cholesterol below</u>

129 mg/l had died, but only half as many of the patients with cholesterol above 223 mg/l.

"High cholesterol is associated with longevity in old people. It is difficult to explain away the fact that during the period of life in which most cardiovascular disease occurs and from which most people die (and most of us die from cardiovascular disease), <u>high cholesterol occurs most often in people with the lowest rate of death</u>. How is it possible that high cholesterol is harmful to the artery walls and causes fatal coronary heart disease, if those, whose cholesterol is the highest live longer than those whose cholesterol is low? To the public and the scientific community I say, "Wake up!" -Uffe Ravnskov, MD, PhD

"We have <u>no evidence</u> that taking a cholesterol lowering medication like a statin will prevent them from getting heart disease." -Elizabeth Nabel, director of the National Heart, Lung, and Blood Institute. Jan, 2008

How to Treat High Blood Pressure Without Drugs

It's estimated that high blood pressure affects 90 percent of Americans at one time or another. Some of the main causes of this condition include lifestyle factors that we have control over such as: eating a high-grain, high-sugar diet, not exercising, stress, and **nerve interference.**

Medically speaking, all cases of high blood pressure are treatable via one way- medication. However, not only does medication NEVER correct the CAUSE of the high blood

pressure, it totes with it devastating and deadly consequences.(shortness of breath, dizziness, flu-like symptoms,
arrhythmia, severe depression progressing to catatonia,
disorientation, memory loss, liver failure, esophagitis, fatal
angioedema and even agranulocytosis, another potential-
ly fatal disorder.) The following information cuts to the true
cause, source, and root of the problem allowing anyone
to achieve freedom from the eternal shackles of modern
pharmaceutica, should they desire.

**"In older individuals with arteriosclerot-
ic vessels, *higher blood pressure is needed* to
maintain adequate blood flow to the kidneys
and other vital organs.** Whatever happened to the
good old days when a *normal systolic pressure was
100 plus your age?* Nevertheless, some senior citizens
will consistently complain of weakness and dizziness if their
blood pressures are lower than the 120/80 value that is
now recommended." -Paul J. Rosch, M.D. Clinical Professor of
Medicine and Psychiatry, New York Medical College

*Exercise: _Regular_ aerobic exercise has been prov-
en to lower blood pressure.

*Drop a Few Pounds: Losing 10 lbs or more
doubles your chance of normalizing your blood pressure
without drugs

*Vitamins C and E: Recent studies have shown that
these antioxidants may help to reduce high blood pressure
by relaxing blood vessels.

*Special 'Atlas Adjustment' Lowers Blood Pressure
Better Than 2 Blood Pressure Medications Combined!
"This procedure has the effect of not one, but two blood-
pressure medications given in combination," reports study

leader George Bakris, MD. "And we saw no side effects and no problems," adds Bakris, director of the University of Chicago hypertension center.

Brain blamed for high blood pressure

High blood pressure is caused by the brain and not the heart, according to a new report which could lead to a radical change in the way the problem is treated. For centuries it has been believed that hypertension is linked to the heart but now that opinion is being challenged. *"Our interests lie in brainstem, or lower part of the brain, and control of blood pressure. We have found evidence that the brainstem is involved in changes over longer timescales. "In hypertensive people there would appear to be an excessive amount of activity in the nerves which connect the brain to the heart and blood vessels causing blood pressure to rise."* http://news.scotsman.com/health.cfm?id=577672007

RISK OF CANCER INCREASING

Researchers recently evaluated data on 114,000 women (ages 22-85) who participated in a California teachers study. The women were free from breast cancer when they enrolled in the study a decade ago. (At that time, the women informed researchers how often and how long they used aspirin and ibuprofen). During a follow up period, some 2400 women were diagnosed with breast cancer. The results of the research were as follows:

1.) Taking _ibuprofen_ every day for at least five years increased a woman's chance of developing breast cancer by <u>50 percent</u>, compared to women who did not regularly take the drug.

2.) <u>Daily use of _aspirin_</u> for five years or more caused a woman's risk of breast cancer to spike by <u>80 percent</u>, compared to non-regular aspirin users. _-Journal of National Cancer Institute, 2005_

If something as seemingly harmless as a little _aspirin_ or _ibuprofen_ can cause a 50-80 % increase in cancer in just 5 years, **then what kind of effect do all the other OTC and prescription drugs have on our body?** Guess what? It's only a matter of time until research proves that **ALL DRUGS (whether pushed or prescribed) CAN AND DO CAUSE CANCER when used to treat symptoms rather than correcting the cause of one's problem.** Is it any mystery why 1 out of 3 people die from cancer in the U.S.? (3rd leading cause of death). We consume 80% of all the drugs in the world! Of course we have a drug problem. However, there's one problem even greater- OUR THINKING! Truly, the "medical model"-that influences your health related decisions- is the #1 cause of death today. Add to that, **SUBLUXATION (blockage of spinal nerves)**, the most devastating thing that will shut down anyone's immune system- and you have 100% certainty for early death by cancer.

If we are ever to truly achieve 100% of our potential for health, healing, and longevity, then we must <u>stop thinking</u>

in terms of pain relief and alternative "treatments". The correct approach to healthcare is the Elevation Health Wellness model: <u>to find and utilize methods that will remove interference to the body's innate healing potential.</u>

CHAPTER 5

"The Healing Diet"

The FIVE FACTORS to determine if this Advanced Diet Plan is Right for *You:*

1. High Triglycerides – If you are a sugar burner and not a fat burner your body will not store or burn fat normally, therefore elevating triglycerides (100 to 135 Normal : > 135 Elevated).

2. High Blood Pressure – Inflammation of the large arteries leads to high blood pressure. Inflammation is controlled by the healing diet.

3. Elevated Glucose / Insulin / Leptin – Once the insulin receptors are burned out, a fasting glucose, insulin, or leptin test will be elevated. Removing all sugar is the only way to heal the insulin receptors.

4. Neurotoxicity – Toxins attached themselves to fat cells and continually elevated leptin. This burns out leptin receptors in the brain leading to leptin

resistance resulting in weight gain that does not respond to exercise and diets.

5. Protein/Fat Genetic Type – Some individuals genetically do better without grains, high fat, or even high protein. This can only be determined by how you feel on a particular diet.

THE FIVE RULES of the HEALING DIET:

The Basic Idea: We must eliminate *all* sugars and *everything* that turns to sugar.

1. NO GRAINS – not even whole, healthy grains!
2. NO SUGARS – this includes hidden sugars (read the ingredients)!
3. NO FRUITS – berries in moderation.
4. Monitor PROTEIN intake – on average 15g per/meal. Larger males and those performing resistive exercise can consume between 20g and 25g per/meal.

    • An egg typically contains 7 grams of protein.
    • A piece of meat the size of a deck of cards typically contains 15 grams of protein.
5. Increase Healthy FATS – 2 to 3 weeks after beginning program. This is the typical time needed to become a fat burner.

FOOD CHOICES
PROTEINS

Choose raw (not roasted for nuts and not pasteurized or homogenized for cheese) grass fed, free-range, cage-free, and no hormone added sources whenever possible. Avoid farm raised and Atlantic fish.

- Cold Water Fish - Salmon, Sardines, Mahi-Mahi, Mackerel etc.
- Eggs
- Cottage Cheese
- Raw Cheeses
- Chicken and Turkey
- Ricotta Cheese
- Beef (grass fed)
- Lamb
- Game Birds - Pheasant, Duck,
- Goose, Grouse
- Whey Protein – Raw Grass Fed
- Venison

FATS

Choose raw (not roasted for nuts and not pasteurized or homogenized for cheese), cold-pressed, grass fed, free-range, cage-free, and no hormone added sources whenever possible. (If Peanut Butter - Valencia Brand).

- Raw nuts & seeds: Almonds, Cashews, Flax, Hemp, Pecans, Pine Nuts, Macadamia, Sesame, Sunflower, Walnuts etc.
- Grass Fed Meat
- Coconut or Flakes

- Cod Liver oil
- Hemp Oil (3 to 1 ratio)
- Olive Oil, Olives
- Flaxseed Oil
- Grape Seed Oil
- Almond Butter
- Avocado
- Real Butter
- Raw Cheeses
- Coconut Milk, Oil, and Spread
- Eggs
- Full Fat Raw Milk
- Full Fat Plain Yogurt
- Lydia's Organics Crackers
- Canned Sardines in Oil or Water
- Cashew Butter

NOTE: AVOID Hydrogenated and Partially Hydrogenated Oils *such as cottonseed oil, soybean oil, and vegetable oils;* Trans Fats *such as margarine and synthetic butters;* Rancid Vegetable Oils *such as corn oil, canola oil, or those labeled simply vegetable oil, located in practically every bread, cracker, cookie, and boxed food.*

HIGH FIBER CARBOHYDRATE (VEGETABLES)

Choose organic when possible. Remember the best carbohydrate choices are vegetables due to high fiber content and low glycemic action.

- Arugula
- Asparagus
- Bamboo Shoots
- Bean Sprouts
- Beet Greens
- Bell peppers (red, yellow, green)
- Broccoli
- Broadbeans
- Brussel Sprouts
- Cabbage
- Cassava
- Cauliflower
- Celery
- Chayote Fruit
- Chicory
- Chives
- Collard Greens
- Coriander
- Cucumber
- Dandelion Greens
- Eggplant
- Endive
- Fennel

- Garlic
- Ginger Root
- Green Beans
- Hearts of Palm
- Jicama (raw)
- Jalapeno Peppers
- Kale
- Kohlrabi
- Lettuce
- Mushrooms
- Mustard Greens
- Onions
- Parsley
- Radishes
- Radicchio
- Snap Beans
- Snow Peas
- Shallots
- Spinach
- Turnip Greens
- Spaghetti Squash
- Summer Squash
- Swiss Chard
- Watercress

CARBOHYDRATE CHOICES IN MODERATION

These carbohydrates can be consumed in small amounts and not on a daily basis.

- Artichokes
- Leeks
- Okra
- Pumpkin
- Tomatoes
- Turnip
- Legumes
- Black Beans
- Adzuki Beans
- Black Beans
- Chick Peas (garbanzo)
- French Beans
- Great Northern

Beans
- Navy Beans
- Kidney Beans
- Lentils
- Mung Beans
- Yellow Beans
- Pinto Beans
- Split Peas
- White Beans
- Lima Beans
- Squash (acorn, butternut, winter)

LOW GLYCEMIC INDEX (GI) FRUIT CHOICES IN MODERATION

Choose organic when possible. If weight loss is a concern eat low glycemic fruit in extreme moderation.

Low GI – Best fruit choice, especially if weight loss is a concern.

- Berries (blackberries, blueberries, boysenberries, elderberries, gooseberries, loganberries, raspberries, strawberries)

LOW FIBER CARBOHYDRATES TO ELIMINATE

These carbohydrates are high and moderate glycemic and turn to sugar very quickly.

- Barley
- Brown Rice
- Buckwheat Groats (kasha)
- Bulgar (tabouli)
- Millet
- Rye
- Semolina (whole grain-dry)
- Steel Cut Oats

- Tapioca
- Whole Grain Breads
- Whole Grain Cooked Cereals
- Whole Grains
- AkMak Crackers
- Ezekiel Bread
- Wasa Crackers
- Whole Grain Tortillas
- Sweet Potato or Yam

COOKING AND EATING TIPS

- If you are not losing weight on this diet. Try reducing your protein intake first.

- If still not losing weight, after protein reduction, your body likely has a toxic interference such as heavy metals and/or biotoxins. Ask your doctor for toxicity testing to identify this interference.

- Removing ALL grains and sugars is easiest when removed completely and at the same time. Your body will adapt to the change quickly and cravings will be eliminated in approximately 1 ½ weeks.

- Eating more frequent meals can minimize symptoms related to glucose and insulin adjustments you may experience when removing grains and sugars from your diet.

- Glutamine will help curb sugar cravings and reduce appetite.

- Doctor recommended protein shake works well as a meal replacement especially while traveling and at work.

- Be sure to drink clean water not tap throughout the day. Reverse osmosis (RO) and/or distilled water is best. Drinking water also reduces appetite.

- Eat protein and good fat with every meal. Raw nuts and seeds are the perfect combination of protein and fat for a snack, if necessary.

TIP 1: COOKING WITH FATS AND OILS – YOU CAN TURN GOOD FATS INTO BAD FATS!

- HIGH HEAT: Use only coconut oil, olive oil, grape seed oil or rice bran oil for frying. The best choice is coconut oil because of its superior flavor when frying food such as chicken or fries. Olive oil, while equally as healthy, tends to make food soggy rather than crispy. A word of caution regarding olive oil: It will turn rancid and become a bad fat when heated above 120° F. If it smokes, it has already turned rancid.

- MEDIUM HEAT: To sauté foods, use sesame oil, rice bran oil, olive oil, grape seed oil, coconut oil or butter.

- BAKING: Butter, coconut oil, sunflower, safflower or olive oil can be used in baking if temperature is less than 325° F. In a hotter oven, use butter, olive oil or coconut butter.

- NO HEAT OILS: Cold-pressed oils such as, flax oil, hempseed oil, sunflower oil, safflower oil and hemp seed oil should not be heated but added to food after it is cooked.

TIP 2: EAT MORE VEGETABLES

- Potatoes are not vegetables, they are tubers.
- If you cook vegetables, lightly steam, but raw is best.
- Some people will do better with more protein and less vegetables and others will do better with more vegetables and less protein, depending on metabolic type (i.e., an Eskimo vs. a Peruvian Indian)
- Listen to your body. Your cravings and energy levels will tell you when you need to adjust or modify your personal plan. However, during the first two weeks while insulin levels are adjusting, you will need to eat more meals a day to feel better.
- Organic is best. If not organic, wash them with distilled vinegar or solution available in health food stores. Use bags to squeeze air out of the vegetables before storing. Sundays seem to be an ideal day to do this for the week.
- Always eat some protein with vegetables (i.e. an egg or piece of chicken, turkey or fish).

TIP 3: ELIMINATING REFINED SUGAR IS CRITICAL

- Refined sugar lowers the immune system.
- Sugar promotes yeast growth.
- One can of soda has 9 to 11 teaspoons of sugar.

- USA: 120 pounds/year per person - 5 pounds/ family (early 1900s)

- Eliminate corn syrup, fructose, honey, sucrose, maltodextrin, dextrose, molasses, rice milk, almond milk, fruit juices, sweetened brown rice syrup, maple syrup, dates, sugar cane, corn, beet, and lactose (the herb *Stevia* is an acceptable sweetener).

- Look at sugar content on all food labels.

- If carbohydrates or sugars are not from above ground vegetables, you should eliminate them (i.e. carrots and potatoes). They will alter insulin levels.

TIP 4: NO MORE GRAINS!

NOTE: It will take several days to lower insulin levels. In the meantime, high insulin levels will cause symptoms such as dizziness, confusion, headaches and a general ill-feeling".

- Eating every two hours can help minimize unpleasant symptoms during this transition.

- 4-6 meals a day is better for weight loss, even after your system adjusts.

- Eating more frequently has shown to normalize blood sugar levels.

- Artificial sweeteners such as NutraSweet, Aspartame, and Sweet & Low, can stimulate carbohydrate and sugar addiction cravings as well as permanent weight loss resistance. © Copyright 2004 Pompa Health Solutions LLC

Part Three

Fat-Burning Fitness

Conditioning your body for full time fat-burning.

"The pain of discipline is far less than the pain of regret."
— Unknown

Most of us have heard the phrase "no pain- no gain." This tends to conjure up in the mind images of hard core, muscle- bound gym freaks thrashing around iron dumb-bells. Obviously, this isn't you or you'd be reading a book on bodybuilding. The fact is that healthy exercise should not be "no pain- no gain," it should be *no pain- no pain.* That's right, healthy exercise should create for you a safe, enjoyable, and rewarding experience.

Just as with any natural science, achieving or main-taining personal fitness must be approached with a strategy. Long before I began my fitness coaching as a cli-ent, I worked out intensively. I just figured pushing harder equaled automatic results. To some degree that was true, but not for long. After a while, I found out that the body plateaus and stops progressing. In addition, not listening to when your body needs rest, causes breakdown, fatigue, injury and discouragement. Simply put, my strategy was guesswork. I knew something was missing, but I needed help to find the right answers. My investment in hiring a coach in this area turned out to yield astronomical returns for me personally as well as helping thousands of people professionally.

As the quest for increasing energy and maintaining a lean physique continues, I find myself honing in on just a few simple principles. Consistency with one's exercise schedule and nutritional habits is paramount to automatic success. Success on cruise control, as I like to describe it, is simply when your day to day routine consists of a few sim-ple, powerful, and regular disciplines. We are all slave to our habits, for better or worse. If this is true, why not make it for the better? We all have a daily ritual of waking up, brushing our teeth, and getting dressed. Why not add one more thing to the list like exercise? It has been said that to cultivate a new habit, it must be repeated for at least 30 days; after that it becomes automatic. After all, there's something to be said for not having to force yourself to do something healthy.

I agree with the wisdom of the ages; that the pain of discipline is far less than the pain of regret. Most of us have a family history full of degenerative disease that claimed the lives of our parents, siblings, and loved ones. I guarantee we can all put our finger on every one of those diseases: Heart disease, Cancer, Diabetes, Thyroid, Kidney disease, Mental Illness....What are you doing now different to avoid the same inevitable fate?

With science and research already having established the fact that 85% of these premature deaths could have been prevented, treated, and cured with PROPER LIFESTYLE, none of us truly has a valid excuse for not "getting in the game."

In the following chapter we will discuss the exact strategies used to engage in an exercise program that will be safe, enjoyable, and literally add years to your life and life to your years.

CHAPTER 1

The Fat-Burning Machine

"All great successes are the triumph of persistence."
— Ralph Waldow Emerson

What most folks wouldn't give to be able to stay lean, trim, energetic, and be able to eat freely all of the time. Sounds too good to be true? Well, almost. While for the majority of us, this would be a far stretch, there are ways to turn the tide in your favor.

There has never been an easier way to create more energy, lose weight, and just feel great than by engaging in regular exercise. If you have ever stayed on a regiment more than a few short weeks (or even days), you have undoubtedly noticed the differences. The question comes into play then as to why more people don't stick with it. There are a few undeniable reasons:

1. "I don't have the time." This turns out to be the exact reason why one should exercise! Lack of exercise

makes it difficult these days for the body to acclimate to stress, control blood sugar, blood pressure, cholesterol, moods, etc...Without exercise, most are doomed to increasing doctors visits, prescriptions, and stays at the hospital. This all adds up to far more time and quality of life lost than that which could be invested to prevent it.

2. "I don't have the energy." This, again, turns out to be the exact reason why one should exercise! Energy is precisely what is abundantly created when engaging in regular exercise properly. The fact that you may have to get up a half- hour earlier in the morning to go for a brisk walk will not leave you more tired. As the day goes on, you will find yourself more energized with greater blood sugar stability. This translates to an increase in focus, increase in productivity, increase in profitability, an increase in self- esteem, an overall healthy mental attitude, and bottom line exponential success. The best part is putting your head on the pillow at night and having no problem falling asleep- and waking well rested to do it all over again the next day!

3. "I can't take the pain." As with anything, when trying something new, you are out of your comfort zone. Mental and physical discomfort is always the first stage to overcome. This is the exact challenge that's necessary to stimulate growth. However, the one gift that God created us all with is the ability to adapt- and survive! Training my body to run 26 miles for the Disney Marathon left an invaluable,

life-long, indelible impression in my heart. That is the fact that you can do anything that you set your heart and mind to, as long as it's done with faith, discipline, and obedience. In today's sedentary, quick fix, prescription happy culture, exercise is no longer merely a recreational option- it's a matter of life and death. The bottom line is that for most of us reading this book right now, this is something that MUST BE DONE in order to prevent disease and early death. Recall that medical research today has proven that 70-85% of most diseases that people are medicated for and dying from, are completely treatable, preventable, and curable with proper lifestyle. This means exercise- FOR LIFE!

CHAPTER **2**

The Fat-Burning Zone

"A professional is a person who can do his best at a time when he doesn't particularly feel like it." — Alistair Cooke

At the time of this writing, I've been exercising regularly now for about 30 years. For the last 10 of those years, I've pursued an increasing interest in aerobic fitness.

When first beginning to run, I didn't think there was much to it; just hit the pavement and work up a sweat. Well, looking back on those days, I can honestly say that I didn't enjoy those workouts very much. I can remember about 3 minutes into my jog, I'd feel this gnawing pain at my side, forcing me to breathe deeply just to keep on. My feet would sometimes hurt. Then weeks later, I'd develop a problem with my knee. Then weeks after that would just get done healing, my back would begin to flare up. It was just one thing after another. Still, I maintained the discipline of following through with my routine, as I realized the overall benefits of keeping a lean physique.

Some years later, my brother Dan was at a nutrition seminar a met a fitness trainer by the name of Stu Mittleman.
Dan got a signed book from him (*Slow Burn) and mailed
it to me. I can remember whizzing through that book like it
was written for me. I digested, absorbed, and utilized every
last bit of Stu's fitness strategies from that book. I figured if
this guy is in the book of records, and recently inducted into
the American ultra- running hall of fame, then I can take it
to the bank! Stu's strategies proved invaluable, as I soon
found my workouts more enjoyable, more effective, and
more energizing. I gained a greater sense of control with my
weight, and overall confidence with my body's fitness level.

The real kicker was when I began teaching these principles in my office workshops. Our workshop attendance
grew 5 fold over the next several months as my patients
returned regularly to continue learning this mind blowing
technology on fitness and nutrition.

I can tell you that the response is always the same.
Whether I am a guest speaker in the community, or in-
house, folks are just blown away by just how much sense
it all really makes. They are inspired and encouraged with
their newfound knowledge, and suddenly become engaged
in something they never thought they'd never have the ability to achieve.

What I learned and what I continue to practice is what I
continue to teach: There are 3 different heart rate zones to
train in. Each has a different effect on the body when sus-
tained for a period of time. By understanding and gaining
control of your heart rate during workouts, you can literally
control just how much fat you will burn.

The MAP zone (mostly aerobic pace): This is
your lowest heart rate zone. It is determined by subtracting

your age from the number 180. So, if your age is 40, you would subtract 180- 40= 140. Then subtract 10 to get your upper MAP limit, and then subtract 20 from that number to get your lower limit. So, if you are 40 years of age your MAP zone would range from 110- 130 beats per minute. Which is to say, by keeping your heart rate within this 20 beat range you will burn fat only during your workout. These workouts are the most healthy, fun, enjoyable, fat- burning, and energizing. Your breathing is more relaxed as you are aware of and in tune with your surroundings and environment. This should be your target zone if you are looking to burn fat, increase energy, balance your blood pressure, cholesterol, blood sugar, and simply prevent sickness and disease, in general.

The MEP zone (mostly efficient pace): This is the middle zone where you now burn sugar and fat. After exceeding the top MAP limit beats per minute range, you enter the sugar burning zone. Going back to our typical 40 year old individual; this would range from 130 to about 140 beats per minute. Your breathing is deeper and your pace is faster, as you begin to train in this more competitive mode.

The SAP zone (speedy aerobic pace): This is your highest heart rate zone where you train at 70 to 80% of your maximum heart rate. At this point, there is only sugar burned for energy. In this extremely competitive mode of training, you are usually only looking for one thing: the finish line- at least that's what I remember. Not a whole lot of fun for most folks at this level of exercise, relatively speaking. I say this from the standpoint of speaking to the general population who rarely or seldom engage in regular exercise. For the majority of us we need to simply and realistically engage in low level and regular exercise routines. The strategies to follow will encompass just that; in addition create a level of health that you probably haven't experienced in decades.

*For more on Stu Mittleman's success training strategies and his ***"Slow Burn"*** book- go to http://www.worldultrafit.com

Fat- Burning Workout Strategy:

Warm Up	*Workout*	*Cool Down*
(5-7 min.)	(15-30 min.)	(5-7 min.)

*Total workout time: 20-40 min.

If your goal is to burn fat, every workout must begin with a warm-up, and end with a cool down. For energy, your body will use one of two sources: Either sugar or fat. You are the one who programs your own body physiology. In other words, you either program your body to burn sugar, or instead teach it to burn fat. Here are a few of the differences:

Burning Sugar:
Short lasting energy
Promotes blood sugar instability
Promotes energy crashing
Promotes fat storage
Promotes diabetes
Promotes lactic acid buildup causing pain and fatigue

Predisposes risk of workout related injury
Promotes build up of free radicals in the body, increasing risk of cancer.

Burning Fat:
Long lasting energy
Promotes blood sugar level stability
Promotes energy increase
Promotes fat burning
Prevents and aids in reversing diabetes
Prevents lactic acid buildup, reducing pain or fatigue
Prevents injury
Prevents free- radical buildup in body

Clearly, we can see the overall health benefits of the fat- burning workout strategy to increase the overall quality of one's life, in general.

The warm up to your workout, in fact, is the exact process that prompts the fat- burning mode. By *gradually* raising your heart rate, you are programming your body to NOT access its sugar stores, but instead, access its fat stores for energy. This is one of the single greatest reasons I see so many people workout, but still struggle with their weight. There tends to be little knowledge, no strategy, and therefore no results. The reason being that their workouts, for the most part, are sugar burning, which ultimately causes FAT- STORAGE! In addition, most folks tend to fall off the wagon very quickly, because such sugar burning workouts cause pain and fatigue, ultimately robbing you of what was supposed to be an energy enhancing, enjoyable experience.

To maintain a lifelong commitment to anything or

anyone, it takes faith, discipline, and obedience- the fruit of which is joy.

The 3 Minute Fat- Burning Version

You may also program your body to burn fat via an alternative strategy, known "as burst training. Recently discovered has been the fat burning effect of high intensity, short duration exercise followed by a 24- 36 hour recovery period. Many studies indicate the effect of high intensity, short duration "burst" or "surge" method of exercise triggering the release of growth hormone following the exercise period. It is the release of Human Growth Hormone that is directly responsible for muscle building and fat burning.

It is important to note that during "classic" aerobic training you are burning mostly fat DURING exercise in the low intensity zone. However, with burst training you, while you may be burning sugar DURING the workout, your body conversely burns more fat during the period of rest (36 hrs.) AFTER the workout, due mainly to the hormonal response from high intensity exercise.

- Rats engaged in a high-intensity sprint training protocol _achieved significant reductions in body fat_ despite the fact that sprint training relied almost completely on carbohydrates as a fuel source
  Hickson, R.C., W. W. Heusner, W.D. Van Huss, D.E. Jac Psaledas. Effects of Dianabol and high-intensity sprint training 8:191-195, \976.

- Found a <u>significant loss in body fat</u> in a group that exercised at a high intensity of 80-90% of Max.

Heart Rate, while no significant change in body fat was found in the lower intensity group which exercised at 60-70% of MHR.

Bryner, R. W., R.C. Tome, I.H. Ullrish, and R.A. Yeater. The effects of exercise intensity on body composition, weight loss, and dietary composition in women. *J. Am. Col.*

What is Burst Training?

- Exercising at 90% to 100% of max effort for 20-30sec. to burn body's stored sugar (glycogen).

- Causes body to burn fat for the next 36 hours to replace your body's vital energy (glycogen) stores.

- Only 3 to 4 sets of 20-30 sec. bursts 3 X week.

- More is not better (must have one day of rest in between workout days).

Basic Workout Plan

- 20 seconds ON
  (Heart rate up to the Training Zone)
- 20 seconds OFF
  (Full recovery time to get heart rate back to bottom of the Training Zone or below)
- 20 seconds ON
- 20 seconds OFF
- 20 seconds ON
- 2 minutes OFF
- Repeat sets as you progress

Lean Muscle Building with Weight Training

Decline Set

- 8-12 repetitions until failure
- Rest 5-6 seconds
- Lower weight 5-20 pounds - 6-8 repetitions until failure
- Rest 5-6 seconds
- Lower weight 5-20 pounds - 6-8 repetitions until failure

Pause Set

- 8-12 repetitions until failure
- Rest 5-6 seconds
- Same weight - repeat until failure
- Rest 5-6 seconds
- Repeat until you cannot do the exercise for more than 1-2 repetitions

The Ultimate Body in 1 hour/week

- 3 burst workouts/week = 12 minutes of exercise with 36 minutes of total elapsed time
- 3 minutes of exercise for each of 8 basic body parts = 24 minutes of total elapsed time
- 1 hour of total time invested/week to get in great shape

The Best Time to Exercise is first thing in the morning on an empty stomach:

- Best compliance
- Raises growth hormone
- Testosterone highest
- Insulin lowest so aids with fat burning
- Turns on metabolism

CHAPTER 3

Eating Fat to Lose fat

"The elevator to success is out of order. You'll have to use the stairs... one step at a time."
— Joe Girard

If you to want to lose fat, you have to eat fat. That's right, no misprint here. At my seminars, I always pause to see the confused looks on everyone's face after that comment. "That doesn't make sense! If I eat more fat won't that make me more fat?" The answer is NO, as long as you eat the *right kind of fat.* Choosing healthy fats, will program your body to lose fat, gain energy, think more clearly, while improving your cholesterol, blood sugar, and blood pressure. How's that for bang for the buck?

You may recall back in elementary school learning that fat has more than twice the calories per kilogram versus protein and carbohydrates. Since 60% of the dry weight of the brain is fat, it turns out that the best source of fuel for your brain and body is good fat. With a healthy metabolism and a diet that approximates about 60% daily caloric intake of these good fats, you are employing a powerful proactive strategy to keep your body in maximum fat burning as well as reducing the risk of Cancer, Heart and Alzheimer's diseases. Remember, good fats are also anti- inflammatory in nature. Saturating your body with these will inevitably reduce the risk of nearly all degenerative diseases that share the common root cause of inflammation.

There is also another factor to be considered. The hormone leptin is what communicates from the fat cells to the brain the actual message that you are full, and when to stop eating. Repeated dietary acidic insults, in addition to elevated insulin levels, causes "leptin resistance." Essentially, this is when the cells become impaired and lose their ability to use the hormone leptin effectively. Ultimately, this translates to more overeating, carbohydrate cravings, tissue breakdown (loss of muscle mass and osteoporosis), fatigue, and FAT- STORAGE! Additionally, this unhealthy cycle leads to high blood pressure, diabetes, depression, and a whole host of degenerative diseases for which most people are medicated for and dying from.

Thus, at the core of any health transformation process must be keeping stable blood sugar levels. Keeping the sugar intake to a minimum will control insulin levels and help to keep you in fat burning vs fat storing. Knowing and choosing the right fuel for meals creates predictable and consistent outcomes for maintaining a healthy body weight and body fat percentage.

What to Increase...

To begin, as well as maintain an alkaline diet and lifestyle, we must first increase our knowledge. However, information without application is hallucination! In order to apply what you are learning, you must now put the rubber to the road. In doing so, we can just start with the just the basic, most fundamental alkalizing foods and elements to add to your diet immediately.

1. Water: Drink roughly 2-3 Liters per day. Specifically, drink 50% of your body weight in oz. Drink between meals not during. Slow gentle saturation. Use a clean, filtered water supply, or spring water (know your alkaline source).
2. Water Rich Vegetables/Greens: Broccoli, cauliflower, cucumbers, onions, sprouts of all kinds, spinach, celery, cabbage, asparagus, and romaine lettuce.
3. Low Sugar Fruits: Lemons, Limes, Tomatoes, Avocados
4. Healthy Fats (Extra Virgin Olive Oil, Fish Oils, Flax Seed Oil, Cod Liver Oil, Coconut oil, Real Butter, Almonds & Walnuts) to name but a few.

By increasing your water consumption, not only are you cleansing your bloodstream and tissues, but also creating a buffer and cellular protection from the damaging effects of internal acids. When cells are well hydrated, your body more readily lets go of unwanted abnormal fat. Additionally, as you increase your daily consumption of good, Omega-3 fats; fish oil, flax oil, and extra virgin olive oil will directly go to work on the cells for repair and regeneration. Thus, by giving your body the fat it needs for healing, it no longer needs to make the extra cholesterol and triglycerides; hence those levels begin to naturally balance out. Also, it no longer needs to hang on to the excess adipose tissue, and so let's go of the hippo hips, and love handles.

Once you create a healthy "internal ecosystem", the cells begin to function properly. Now we have proper polarity allowing the cells to move more rapidly through the bloodstream, carrying more oxygen to the tissues, thus creating more energy. Amazingly, as well, when you eat good fat foods like avocados and almonds, your hunger is satisfied. That's because even when you eat a small amount of food that's high in fat, it allows your brain to hear the "no longer hungry" message. The restored integrity to the body cells, enhances leptin hormone production, and decreases leptin resistance and the disease of obesity commonly associated with it.

Little things make a BIG difference.

By simply adding the above essentials to your daily diet, you will begin to notice immediate changes in your energy, weight, and body- fat. The key is consistency. I can tell you, beyond a shadow of a doubt, if you do this daily, then it will become a habit. As you sow a habit, you reap your character. As you sow in your character, you reap your destiny. We become slave to our habits- for better or worse. If you become slave to good habits, then your success is virtually on autopilot!

CHAPTER 4

Proper Hydration

"Nothing needs reforming so much as other people's habits." — Mark Twain

One of the easiest and most effective ways to increase your energy, mental clarily, focus, lose body fat, and prevent degenerative disease is to simply drink enough water. There is so much to be said about this topic, that many physicians have written volumes of books and have dedicated their entire career focusing on the healing properties of water. The fact that dehydration is a dangerous and deadly condition to the human body is common sense. However, the silent and gradual process of dehydration makes us susceptible to treat the resulting symptoms in a blind sighted fashion.

70% of your body is made up of water. Next to oxygen, this is the most primary essential for life. The bloodstream needs water as part of the medium for communication and transportation of blood cells, fat cells, and hormones that are conducive to normal function and healing in the body. Every system in your body depends on water.

Lack of water causes a lack of protection from the acid diet and lifestyle. Just as the body uses good fat to repair, regenerate and protect the cells, so does water. It creates a medium and buffer as a means of protection for the blood cells, maintaining proper blood pH.

In my workshops, I always challenge the participants to simply increase their daily intake of water and watch what happens. After applying this simple discipline consistently, I have never had an individual report anything less than an overall feeling of increased vitality and well being. The results are almost immediate for those who are willing to convert this simple discipline into a daily habit.

These folks become quickly addicted to a good thing; carrying a liter bottle to work or school and gently sipping between their meals a full liter, totaling between 2 and 3 liters per day. The rule of thumb is to consume approximately half your bodyweight in fluid ounces of clean, pure water each day. So, if you weighed 200 lbs, then you'd be looking to consume around 100 oz. per day. This converts to a little more than 3 liters. Immediate benefits include:

- Improve Your Energy
- Increase Your Mental and Physical Performance
- Remove Toxins & Waste Products from your body
- Keep Skin Healthy and Glowing
- Help You Lose Weight
- Reduce Headaches and Dizziness
- Allow for proper Digestion
- Help to keep you more Alkaline

The findings of a six-year study of more than 20,000 healthy men and women aged 38-100 in the May 1, 2002 American Journal of Epidemiology found that women who drank more than five glasses of water a day were 41% less likely to die from a heart attack during the study period than those who drank less than two glasses. The protective effect of water was even greater in men.

Water is a natural appetite suppressant, so developing a good water drinking habit can be a long-term aid in achieving and maintaining a healthy weight.

Water is especially important for pregnant women and nursing mothers. For athletes and work-out fanatics, drinking water reduces cardiovascular stress and improves performance. And, since water reduces body temperature, it makes the whole exercise process safer and more effective.

Water is also an important "healing tool" for people with a history of kidney stones. Since water dissolves calcium in the urine, downing at least 8 glasses daily reduces the risk of stone formation. Drinking water is also valuable in preventing urinary tract infections in both men and for women, flushing impurities out of the system.

Even mild dehydration makes you more susceptible to viruses. For someone with an immune system compromised from cancer, water is a powerful weapon in war on colds and other illnesses. Water helps you recover more quickly from illness.

When your body is hydrated, drainage from allergies and colds doesn't stick and collect in your throat and lungs, and your cough is more "productive". Even cold sores that appear on the lips are minimized by drinking water because those eruptions tend to favor dry areas on the body.

The Benefits of Water

Is drinking so much water really necessary?

"Absolutely," says Cleveland Clinic nutritionist Andrea Dunn. "Almost every cell in your body needs water to function properly. Many of the patients I see don't drink enough water. They aren't dehydrated, but they aren't drinking as much water as they should -- especially considering how much your body needs."

The human body, which is made up of between 55 and 75 percent water (lean people have more water in their bodies because muscle holds more water than fat), is in need of constant water replenishment.

Your lungs expel between two and four cups of water each day through normal breathing - even more on a cold day. If your feet sweat, there goes another cup of water. If you make half a dozen trips to the bathroom during the day, that's six cups of water. If you perspire, you expel about two cups of water (which doesn't include exercise-induced perspiration).

A person would have to lose 10 percent of her body weight in fluids to be considered dehydrated, but as little as 2 percent can affect athletic performance, cause tiredness and dull, critical thinking abilities. Adequate water consumption can help lessen the chance of kidney stones, keep joints lubricated, prevent and lessen the severity of colds and flu and help prevent constipation.

How do you know if you are drinking enough water?

A good test is to look at your urine. If it's clear, you're

doing a good job of staying hydrated. But if it's intense yellow or gold, you probably need to drink more water.

Even mild dehydration - as little as a 1 percent to 2 percent loss of your body weight - can sap your energy and make you tired. Dehydration poses a particular health risk for the very young and the very old. Signs and symptoms of dehydration include:

- Excessive thirst
- Fatigue
- Headache
- Dry mouth
- Little or no urination
- Muscle weakness
- Dizziness
- Lightheadedness

Proper Hydration Recommendations

1. You are naturally thirsty i.e. "dehydrated" in the morning. To help your body flush out the toxins it has been processing all night, take advantage of this thirst to get a "leg up" on your daily water requirements by drinking a glass of water first thing.

2. Don't wait until you're thirsty to have a drink – you are already dehydrated if you feel thirsty.

3. Set a timer to remind yourself to establish a habit of drinking water and keep a bottle of water with you at all times.

4. Compensate for diuretics- thieves that rob water

from your body. If you drink coffee, tea, or sodas with caffeine, you'll need to drink a few extra glasses of water to make up for the water that these diuretic beverages "leech" from your system.

5. Though uncommon, it's possible to drink too much water. Drinking excessive amounts can overwhelm your kidneys' ability to get rid of the water. This can lead to hyponatremia, a condition in which excess water intake dilutes the normal amount of sodium in the blood. People who are older, who have certain medical conditions such as congestive heart failure and cirrhosis, or who are taking certain diuretics are at higher risk of hyponatremia.

6. A trace mineral deficiency can be a causative factor for dehydration. Solar dried or air dried pink salt from PR labs is a mix of Mediterranean and Hawaiian sea salt. Because their production process does not utilize a super heating process (over 1000 degrees) to dry it, the ultimate benefit is that the product retains over 90 different trace minerals necessary for hydration. Recall hydration and body fat percentage is typically inversely proportional. The more well hydrated you are, the more willing the body is to let go of unwanted/ unhealthy fat.

Part Four

CHAPTER 1

Houston Control

"To accomplish great things, we must not only act but also dream. Not only plan but also believe." — Anatole France

When a sperm and egg unite, there is fertilization. The cells then continue to multiply and divide until the 18th day after conception when we see the beginnings of the central nervous system. The central nervous system consists of the brain, spinal cord, and spinal nerves. Amazingly, it has been my experience that the average person was not even aware that life begins with your nervous system. In other words, you don't have a heart, lungs, liver, spleen, kidneys, or any other organs exist until the brain and nerve system are formed and in place. The reason being is that when God breathes life into a living being there must be a vessel or a conduit to serve as a means of communicating the intelligence He has placed within us. It is that Innate or in-born intelligence that uses the nerve system to coordinate the development of all organs, cells, and tissues within the fetus, as well as controlling all function and healing in the newborn and adult.

If we cut the nerves going to your eyes, would you see or go blind? If we cut the nerves going to your teeth, what would happen? They would rot and eventually fall out. If all the nerves going to your heart were completely severed, you would almost immediately die. The reason for this is that the nerve supply brings LIFE to the parts of the body. And wouldn't it make sense that if something brings LIFE to a part of the body, then it also brings HEALING? In essence, your nerve system controls ALL function and healing everywhere in the body- at all times.

Think of all the times you went to your medical physician for your annual checkup: They checked your blood pressure, cholesterol, blood sugar, prostate exam, mammogram, etc... But when they find something wrong, do they check the one system that controls all function and healing? No. They simply treat the effects with drugs. High Blood pressure- no problems take this. Insulin resistant diabetes- take that. Headaches- take 2 of these and call me in the morning. Prescriptions are very effective at masking symptoms, but NEVER correct the cause of your heath problem. If all you do is treat effects to the neglect of correcting the CAUSE of the problem, that person will be on medication for the rest of their lives (exactly as the pharmaceutical companies would have it).

The key to correcting the cause of one's health issues is to locate and correct THE CAUSE of interference to the proper function and innate healing ability of the body.

Remember, God put the most amazing healing power in your Nerve System. That power must flow from the brain, down the spinal cord, and out over the nerves to animate every cell, organ, and tissue in your body. When this brain- body communication path is clear and unobstructed, you have a condition known as health. However, if there is any obstruction or blockage to this path, we have communication breakdown between the brain and body, resulting in sickness and disease. The primary question to be asked then is what could CAUSE this INTERFERENCE?

Vertebral Subluxation

Vertebral Subluxation is a condition where one or more of the spinal bones lose their normal position relative to the bone above and below. This creates an occlusion producing pressure on the spinal cord, and/ or spinal nerves. This pressure then creates a blockage or interference to the normal nerve supply from the brain, thus resulting in sickness and disease at the end of those nerve fibers.

Therefore, if there's blockage to the nerves going to the heart, you eventually develop a heart problem. Block the nerves going to the pancreas, and soon enough will develop diabetes. Shut down the nerves going to the kidneys, and eventually the kidneys will shut down. In my experience, anytime I have had a man present to me with a case of prostate cancer, or prostate enlargement, the X-rays have clearly demonstrated damage and long term blockage of the lumbar nerve roots that feed out to the prostate- 100% of the time, in every case.

As a matter of fact, any time I have ever had a patient present to me with ANY DISEASE of ANY KIND, I have always been able to trace it back to spinal damage and nerve blockage AT THE EXACT LEVEL of the spine where the nerves exit to feed that organ or part of the body. These types of findings are typical and correlate with medical study findings from a 1921 research project conducted in Dresden, Germany called "The Windsor Autopsy Studies." Freshly frozen cadavers were used to clearly illustrate the devastating, degenerative effects of the vertebral subluxation condition. They found a nearly 100% correlation between the disease a patient died from and the damaged spinal nerves involved.

Vertebral Subluxation can cause virtually any disease or health condition known to mankind when it is rooted in the central nerve system. I have seen it cause cancer, heart disease, diabetes, depression, kidney and thyroid disease, blindness, and deafness, to name a few.

In fact, the first patient to ever have a spinal subluxation scientifically detected and corrected was Harvey Lillard, a deaf janitor, in Davenport, Iowa. On September 18th 1895, Dr. D.D. Palmer examined a large bump protruding on the neck of Lillard. He determined that if this bone out of place produced the deafness, then reducing the bump would reduce or correct the condition. His theory tuned out to be correct, as Harvey Lillard received his hearing back after his first adjustment.

With over 600 new sets of spinal x-rays I take each year, I can confidently say that there is absolutely no way for an individual to have hope for a healthy future, where there continues to be neglect for the spine and central nerve system. This statement is based on physical laws of the human body, and not merely my opinion.

Hippocrates, the father of modern medicine, said "look well to the spine for the cause of disease." By the way, his was a drugless approach, as well.

Causes of Vertebral Subluxation

From the womb to the tomb, we are all subject to stresses, slips, falls, and traumas that suddenly or progressively cause displacement of spinal vertebrae. In 1969, Dr. Abraham Towbin, a Harvard pediatric neurologist set out to discover the cause of neonatal spinal cord injuries. He found that in over 80% of sudden infant death syndrome case autopsied, the cause of death was attributable to pressure on the brainstem via spinal subluxation. (1) This mechanism of injury is caused by pulling the baby by the head too forcefully out of the birth canal during delivery. This is substantiated by the fact that the brainstem and upper cervical spine controls one's breathing, blood pressure and immune system. When I see this pattern on any patients x-ray, whether newborn or adult, I immediately become concerned. Most of these children have already developed asthma, allergies, ear infections, and related immune deficiency illnesses. Adults typically present with chronic headaches, high blood pressure, tiredness and fatigue, dizziness, sinus and allergy problems, nervousness and depression, and sometimes dizziness, to name a few.

Among other causes of vertebral subluxation in children would be learning to walk, rolling off a bed and landing on the neck the wrong way, or falling off of a bike or out of a tree or a swing. Additionally, most kids (and adult weekend warriors) are subject to sports impacts and injuries. Nearly everyone has been involved in at least one motor vehicle accident (the average is 3 in a lifetime). Sleeping on a bad mattress, over time, can cause the equivalent damage of sustaining several auto accidents to the spine. Slip and fall injuries at home, work, or elsewhere are very typical presenting cases I see. Then, of course, you have the epidemic work environment today of sitting at a computer looking down all day causing chronic problems in the neck and upper back. These are just a few of the most common causes of vertebral subluxation.

A Different Healing Perspective

At over 20,000 visits seen annually out of my clinic, you can bet I see a range of all types of people presenting with every kind of sickness or disease known to mankind.

As a chiropractor, my focus is much more important than simply treating one's symptom, ailment, or disease. More importantly, it is to locate and correct THE CAUSE of that person's illness. The technology and testing we use in our clinic is directed at pinpointing with precision accuracy the exact location of any blockage or damage to the spinal cord or spinal nerves.

Infrared thermal spinal scanning technology, along with digital x-rays enable us to detect any blockage, damage or pinching of the nerves that exit from the spine. Regardless of the condition a patient presents with, we will always order these diagnostic tests. The reason? Very simply, in order to determine if we can help someone, we need to determine the CAUSE of their condition. If the cause is in the spine, and IT IS still within means of correction, then we can assume that individual will respond well and heal.

Whether the condition is high blood pressure, diabetes, cancer, radiating neck and back pain with sciatica, or thyroid disease; the neurological testing that is done will be to determine the presence of vertebral subluxation that has caused or precipitated that disease.

Once confirmed, the x-rays are analyzed, thoroughly studied, and patient then recommended a course of corrective care. Gentle, specific chiropractic adjustments are given to correct vertebral alignment and restore proper nerve supply to all damaged tissues and organs.

If an individual has developed diabetes solely due to a blockage of proper nerve supply, and I open up the blockage- that person heals. If the cause of an individual's high blood pressure is a misaligned C1 vertebrae exerting pressure on the brainstem and spinal nerves, and I find and correct the cause of this with a specific scientific chiropractic adjustment- that person heals. If a child presenting with asthma is found to have subluxation at the level of T1 on x-ray where the nerves feed out to the lungs, and we restore proper nerve supply- that person heals. These are only a few case examples mentioned of the many that I see on a daily basis.

Most of the people who present to my office with these conditions on medications are able to reduce their prescription usage, or completely get off. Not because I tell them to throw their drugs in the trash can, but because they frequently return to their medical physicians for follow up testing that confirms the restoration of normal physiological function, and no longer warrants prescription drug usage. Therefore, their own doctors take them off the drugs.

In our clinic we are scientific with a vengeance. We do not give quick "pops", "cracks", or "fixes" simply for pain relief on the spot. We carefully and thoroughly review any and all x-rays, scans, and test results before administering any care to any patient whatsoever.

Additionally, before accepting any cases for care, a patient must demonstrate a certain level of commitment to responsibility for their own health and healing by attending through a new patient orientation. This process not only lays the foundation for their immediate healing, but the roadmap to wellness and prevention thereafter. I consider it a blessing and a gift to my patients to be able to teach them how to prevent illness and disease from affecting their family, thus enabling them to stay off of medications, out of doctors offices, and out of hospitals. This ultimately saves them time, money, and future emotional trauma.

Prevention: The Only True Cure

Stephen Covey is quoted with saying "start with the end in mind." I tell all patients this from day one: Your spine requires maintenance. It always has. If something requires maintenance and you neglect it, you WILL develop problems. Not sometimes or maybe, but rather just a question of when. If you don't brush your teeth, you get cavities. If you don't keep the oil in your car engine, it'll shut down.

Your spine and nerve system both work in the same fashion. Because we are all subject to daily stresses and strains, the spine requires regular check- ups to detect and correct any spinal nerve interference BEFORE it causes any pain, sickness, or disease. When the average adult presents to our office without ever having a proper neurologically based spinal checkup, you can bet we find problems the majority of the time. That's like going to the dentist the first time at age 40 without ever having brushed your teeth.

Therefore, most folks who start care in our office do so

with the idea of first and foremost MAKING UP FOR LOST TIME, getting the spine stabilized, corrected, and finally (and most importantly) MAINTAINED for life.

The benefits of maintenance/ wellness care go far beyond preventing unwanted everyday aches and pains. Since beginning my practice career in 1993, I have found that individuals and families that have stayed under regular wellness care are some of the healthiest people on the planet. They are on little or no prescription medication. They make fewer trips to the doctor or pediatrician. They pay lower insurance premiums, and rarely get the flu or chronic colds.

Imagine what life would be like living at your God given health potential. This book has given you more than all of the tools and knowledge necessary for massive change and transformation. All that is needed from here is discipline and consistency. May God bless you in your pursuit of excellence!

CHAPTER 2

Patients Speak Out

"Somebody should tell us, right at the start of our lives that we are dying. Then we might live life to the limit, every minute of every day. Do it! I say. Whatever you want to do, do it now! There are only so many tomorrows."
— Michael Landon

My Life Changed by Chiropractic Care

Dear Reader:

It was about 2 years ago that I entered the office of Champion Chiropractic and knew that my life would be changed forever.

I lived in a small island in the Caribbean known as the Commonwealth of Dominica, where no chiropractic care is available. At the age of 14 years old, I fell down a hole about 21 FT deep and injured myself, which began all my problems.

At the age of 22 years of age I was diagnosed with

migraine headaches, other illnesses and very asthmatic. I also began having occasional back pain that was relieved with either Tylenol or Ibuprofen.

After graduating from nursing school where I received my registered nursing degree, I began having sharp pains down my legs and was told that I was having sciatica. Once again I began using painkillers and muscle relaxants to relieve the pain. Three months later, while helping a patient, my back suddenly went into spasms that caused me to be unable to do anything else for the rest of the night.

For the next 10 years I went in and out of hospitals, tried doctor after doctor and even traveled to the neighboring island of Guadeloupe several times, each time seeing a different doctor in search of an answer to my problem. However, I was told over and over again that nothing was surgically wrong with my back and that I was imagining it all. One doctor even told me that I should have psychotherapy. Due to my illness, I finally was asked to take a medical retirement from my job because of my being sick so often. I reluctantly complied to do so at the age of 34.

After 9 years of suffering and trying to raise two children, my world began to fall apart, even with the full support of my husband and family members. I felt like life was not worth living anymore, and I even became angry with God, not knowing that all the time he had a plan for my life.

Somewhere deep within me I felt that I needed to try one last time. I surfed the internet and chose one of the top 3 neurosurgeons in the US. After visiting this physician it was then that I knew that it was finally over. He told me the same thing the others did that "you have nothing surgically wrong with your back." He indicated that I should continue with my physical therapy and he even recommended that I attend a pain control clinic.

Upon my return to Miami after visiting the neuro-surgeon, my brother who had been telling me about a Chiropractor said to me "okay, you have tried everything, it won't hurt to try the Chiropractor.

I must confess that I was skeptical at first and did not believe in Chiropractic care which was the reason why I did not take my brother's advice when he told me to see Dr. Yachter before going to another medical doctor. I finally agreed and the next day we went to the office of Dr. David Yachter. The staff was very warm and there was concern in the doctor's eyes when he spoke to me.

After looking at my x-rays, which were the same ones that the neurosurgeon saw, without telling him what was going on with me, Dr. Yachter told me every symptom that I was experiencing. I could not believe my ears. He reassured me that I was not psychologically ill, and that my problem was real. The only thing that kept me from crying was the fact that I was with a total stranger. I could not take the full course of the treatment then, because after one month of adjustments I had to return home. During that month however, I was convinced that the answer to my problem lies within that form of treatment. In one month, I was able to do many things I was unable to do before, but the most dramatic change was the fact that I did not need painkillers during that month.

One and a half year later, I returned to Miami to have the chiropractic care. I arrived there in a wheelchair and drugged with painkillers and muscle relaxants. I returned to Dr. Yachter's office the following day and began my care.

Today, I must say that I am a walking miracle. It has been almost nine months since I started having there adjustments, and during that time I have been off pain medication. I can now exercise and do most of the things I used to do. The natural curve in my neck is being restored, and the double scoliosis has been corrected. Most of all the sleepless nights are over, because I do not have to take drugs to sleep, and I have gotten my life back. Thanks first of all to God, then to Dr. Yachter without whom I would have been dead before I became 40 years of age.

I had to leave my husband and children to come to the United States of America to receive this type of care. Today, I know it was the sacrifice, and I am now ready to return home to be the wife, mother and nurse that I have always wanted to be.

Please do not wait to be in the position I was in when all else have failed to try Chiropractic care. You are more fortunate than I was because you have the Chiropractors more accessible than other people do in the islands. Do not wait to start having symptoms before seeing Chiropractic care. Please make it a part of your life as much as you do your dentist, primary care physician and other physicians. These doctors take care of your other functions of your body, but chiropractors take care of your source of life, which is your central nervous system. When you receive chiropractic care you will find that you spend less and less money on medical doctors and drugs, and you will have more time to do the things that are important to you. Due to subluxation you are slowly dying and you don't even know it. Only chiropractic care can add more years to your life. I know because I am a living proof of it.

I know that there are many chiropractors in America, but I can only speak of one and that is Dr. David Yachter. He and his staff are very loving and caring and their primary concern is to see their patients function at optimal health. They will do all they can in their power to see that you achieve that goal. The power workshops are also eye openers as they enlighten your mind as to what is actually happening in your body and world. Give yourself a treat. Please call Champion Chiropractic today for an appointment at (954) 472-6002. I know that you will not regret it because I don't.

I will be eternally grateful to God for leading me to Dr. David Yachter and his staff.

A Grateful Client,
Julia L.

ﻮﻮﻮ

"My health problems before receiving chiropractic care consisted of high blood pressure and I was heavily medicated. I was skeptical before starting chiropractic care because I thought that it was only for people with back problems or for someone who has been in an accident. It made a lot of sense to me with my scientific background. I immediately saw its relevance in solving my problem. Now I feel a lot more energized. My breathing and my blood flow are much better. I have not taken any blood pressure medication for about 7 weeks now and my blood pressure has settled in to the normal range. After becoming a patient of Dr. Yachter's I have told all of my friends and family that they need to have their spine checked. This can help them discover any nerve blockage they may have."

-Ricardo M.
October 22, 2008

"Prior to chiropractic care, I had lower back pain and pain in my right shoulder. It affected my life in many ways. It was difficult for me to walk sometimes. In addition, it was painful getting out of bed. Before chiropractic care and the orientation, I was a bit skeptical. After chiropractic care and after attending the orientation, I am more confident in your services and ability to improve my health. Since chiropractic care, all of the issues I experienced with my back pain and shoulder have been improved dramatically. I am able to walk better and my eye sight has improved. I went to my eye doctor and my vision improved from 25/40 to 25/25. I would share my health improvements and experiences with my family and friends. I would highly recommend your services to anyone."

-Pauline Brewster
July 24, 2008

"My health problems before starting with chiropractic care consisted of pulling on my right side, unable to sleep and my back was totally out of alignment. Before beginning chiropractic care, I knew it was helpful but I did not realize how critical it was to good health. I am definitely a believer in chiropractic corrective care! Since my very first adjustment, I have been able to sleep through the night and I have less headaches. I can also feel less tension in my body. I have told my family and friends about the things I have learned from Dr. Yachter and how life changing it is!

-Harriette H.,
October 9, 2008

꒰꒰꒰

"I had a history of colon and liver cancer and male pattern baldness. Before starting care at Champion Chiropractic, I had never felt the need to seek the services of a chiropractor since I thought that those services were only used for back related problems. Now that I have been a patient of Dr. Yachter's for about 2 years, it has been a new revelation on how God created the body to function perfectly. My barber just recently asked me what I was doing to make my hair grow back? I gave her business cards from Dr. Yachter's office and explained his treatment program. To God be the glory! I have told all my family and friends about Champion Chiropractic. I even tell strangers that I meet about how God is using the method to heal people's needs."

-Alphonso B.,
September 16, 2008

ᴊᴊᴊ

"I had many issues before receiving chiropractic care. I was experiencing constant chronic pain in my neck and shoulders. At times the inability to sleep or be comfortable was overwhelming. Sitting, standing, laying flat and lifting small objects was unbearable. Before chiropractic care, my fear was paralysis and dislocation of joints. Honestly, I do not like strangers touching me. After coming in to the office to begin care, I thought the orientation was very informative. I was very comfortable with the chiropractic care due to the professionalism of the doctor. My health has definitely improved since starting care. I am able to run errands for an extensive period of time without experiencing pain in my neck, back and legs. I have the ability to sit at the dining room table and read, pray, listen to music, plan events and watch television in the den with my family. I have told my family and friends about chiropractic care. It gave me a sense of renewed living without discomfort, pain and freedom to live a normal and more productive life. My headaches are gone after just one chiropractic adjustment!"

-Sandra W,
September 26, 2008

ᴊᴊᴊ

"Before coming to the chiropractor, I was having trouble sleeping and did not have much energy. For me, the chiropractor was just for people who had back problems.

After the evaluation, I came to realize how important it is to take care of your spine and have good habits. Everything I learned makes sense!

After coming to chiropractic care, I am sleeping and breathing much better. I have more energy and my posture is better as well. I now recommend chiropractic care with Dr. Yachter to all of my friends and family. In his office you don't just get an adjustment, you learn how to improve your health!"

-Adriana T.
June 19, 2008

ﾉﾉﾉﾑ

"Before starting chiropractic care, my energy level was very low. By mid-afternoon I was always tired and edgy. I suffered from pain in my lower back and on my left side from my hip all the way to my toes. I had leg cramps at night and tingling sensations in my fingers and toes. My blood pressure was high. I also had pains in my neck and arms. I was not able to hold my head up to do any task; if I did I would get dizzy. Before chiropractic care and before attending the orientation my feelings we positive. I heard Dr. Yachter on the radio and I called to make an appointment. That was the best decision I have ever made! After starting care, my feelings became more positive. I was impressed by the nerve scan and I learned that chiropractic care was not only for pain relief. I no longer have difficulty holding my head up to do tasks, attacks of dizziness are less frequent, my energy level has improved and I am no longer edgy or nervous as before. I feel much better physically and emotionally! I would tell my family and friends about chiropractic care. It is a good alternative to main stream healthcare. Get your spine adjusted, remove subluxations, remove pressure from spinal nerves, improve nutrition and let Gods healing flow to all organs thereby preventing disease and early death. Give chiropractic a try, you will be glad you did! God continue to bless Dr. Yachter and the Champion Chiropractic Team!!!"

-Jasmine W.
June 9, 2008

⌒⌒⌒

"Before receiving chiropractic care, I use to urinate frequently during the day and at night. Every morning I would get up tired because I would get up at least three times during the night to use the bathroom. I had a positive feeling about chiropractic care before coming to your office because I have a great interest in the field of alternative medicine. After coming to the orientation, I was more convinced that chiropractic care would be the best choice for treating my medicals ailments and preventing the same illness also. Since I began chiropractic care, I have been sleeping better at nights and I don't have that urinary problem anymore. I recommend chiropractic care to everyone because it saves lives, whereas medications destroy lives."

-Leona E.
June 5, 2008

"Before seeking chiropractic care I had just been di-agnosed with spinal stenosis and was experiencing very painful symptoms from the nerves involved. I was always tired and had extremely low energy. I always believed in chiropractic care and even had received some years ago. But it was very different then what it is now. I usually just got adjusted "when needed". Today the knowledge and tech-nology has come a long way. Total healthcare is involved! More information is available about healthy eating; deadly toxins and harmful drugs prescribed to so call make us "well". Since being treated at Champion Chiropractic, I have almost no symptoms from the stenosis, have been able to get off my blood pressure medication and my ener-gy has increased. I have a general sense of well being now. I've learned a new tool for greater health care. I will tell all my friends and family of my experience with chiropractic care. If they want to live better and longer chiropractic care will enable them to do that. Thanks be to God!"

-Rene C.
February 1, 2009

"It was the third time in my life that a watershed event was to happen. And for the third time it was Chiropractically life-changing!

The First:

I was about 7 years old & away at summer camp. We were swimming in this beautiful lake that had a slide located near its shore. Apparently, I was the only one who didn›t know there was a round metal tub sunk beneath the end of the slide. It had a fairly sharp lip on its perimeter. Head first I slid down & ostensibly cracked open the top of my head on impact. A fractured skull & thirty stitches later, the Camp Dr. couldn›t understand how I survived. For thirty some odd years thereafter, I would suffer from headaches, sometimes on a daily basis, sometimes from migraines, but always debilitating to various degrees.

Dr. David Yachter, my oldest son, was in his first term at Life Chiropractic College. At home, during his first semester break he asked if he could try an adjustment that might help my chronic headaches. It only took a few seconds, but the Occipital lift, which substantially moved my head off its atlas, gave me a rush & then a wonderful feeling of calm. My neck had been subluxated all those years. Over time when David came home from School, I›d get another adjustment & gradually the headaches would disappear. I no longer have headaches. It was Chiropractically life-changing.

The Second:

April 2001, it was a bike accident. Riding my twelve speed around the development where I live, for whatever reason, at about 20 miles per hour, I wound up flying over the handle bars. Landing squarely on my face, with the exception of my jaw, most of my facial bones were shattered. By all accounts my neck and spinal column should have broken as well... I would have been left a paraplegic. But, they were intact. The only explanation was that for ten years I had been receiving Chiropractic adjustment almost on a weekly basis. As a result, my neck & spinal column were supple enough to absorb the enormous impact. It took six months after major surgery, but I healed. I have almost no residual effects. It was Chiropractically life-changing.

The Third:

Almost twelve years ago my blood tests showed some serious problems. My Triglycerides were 381, Cholesterol at 275 & weight about 230 pounds. For me, these numbers were very dangerous to say the least. Interestingly, I had neither reaction nor response from the medical Dr. who called for the blood work, not even a phone call! About six months ago I again had a blood workup. This time my Triglycerides showed 263, Cholesterol @ 168 and weight of 225 pounds. A little better, or so I thought. I sent these numbers to my younger son, Dr. Daniel Yachter, which sent shivers down his spine. He immediately called & we spoke for an hour & a half, discussing their significance and implications. Stressing the fact that I was a prime candidate for a heart attack, or even worse, a stroke, Daniel pushed hard for me to go on a "Healing Diet «. I was ready, and took his advice to heart. Three months after I began the «Healing Diet», I again had a blood workup. The numbers showed, that the "Healing Diet « works and works well. In addition to my Triglycerides dropping to 57, HDL to 87, LDL 101, my weight dropped a totally unexpected 25 pounds! The rest of my vitals were well within the normal range. But that isn›t the best of it. After the first three months of dieting I stopped using Prilosec (heart burn medication) and as of this writing I have been off Synthroid (Thyroid medication) for several months. For the first time in 34 years I am completely drug free! I am still on the «Healing Diet», and once again it has been Chiropractically life-changing

PS Daniel now says that at 68, I am starting to grow younger. If, with Chiropractic care and use of the « Healing Diet « , a body-wide regeneration of healthy cells can be achieved , then   I believe my son the Chiropractor may indeed have found the fountain of youth!"

Sid Y.
2-10-09

It was in October of 2006 that a medical check-up revealed that I had high blood pressure! In fact, as I was sitting waiting for the nurse to proceed with an EKG the blood pressure reading was so high that she literally rushed out of the room and a few moments later returned with a second person to give me a thorough check. Then announced that she would not allow me on the treadmill due to the blood pressure reading which was around 164 over 144. I was shaken, to say the least. I was instructed to visit my doctor immediately. **After another examination by my** family doctor I was placed on a medication that was more mild, thinking that this would take care of my condition. **But that medication didn't work effectively,** so I returned a second time to my family doctor and was prescribed a second medication, much stronger than the first. This medication worked and my blood pressure came down to acceptable limits. **I was told that losing weight, more exercise and taking my medicine regularly would** help me maintain a normal blood pressure reading and that in time, perhaps but not guaranteed, I would be able to get off of the medicine all together. That didn't happen. It was in March of 2008 that I met Dr. Yachter through my Pastor in Miami, Florida. Dr. Yachter began adjustments immediately. After trying several times before to just quit the medication without success, three months of chiropractic adjustments and I am completely off all medications. As of this writing the last three days of my blood pressure was as follows: 126 over 73 with 48 BPM, 124/76 with 60 BPM and this morning 128/80 with 54 BPM.

-Steve B.,
July 2008

ﬧﬧﬧ

I suffer from diabetes and the affect it has had on my daily life is little other than having to make sure to squeeze in time from my already busy schedule to do my exercises in order to keep my blood sugar at a safe level. I was often feeling fatigued and suffered from allergies. I never really thought about chiropractic being of any benefit to a diabetic. I had no idea that it would benefit my overall health to see a chiropractor. After seeing Dr. Yachter for several months my blood sugar was down by an average of 30-40 points and it even maintains hours after a meal and my allergies were gone. I was no longer feeling tired and it seemed that when I did my usual stretches I could reach my toes much better than before. I still have to exercises because that is always important. I am also in much better cardiovascular health. The Holy Spirit willed me to do this and I will never look back and regret it. I fell that this experience has definitely had a positive effect on my life. If you have any health problems you should see a chiropractor first and check that your spine is in line and that all of your organs are getting the juice and signals they need from your brain.

-Gordon C.,
9/04

ﻼﻼﻼ

Before receiving chiropractic care, I was on 6 different medications for asthma, high blood pressure, cholesterol, allergies, a skin condition and for my heart. My breathing was limited. I wheezed with the slightest bit of exertion and I had to sleep sitting up.

Before coming to this office, I was seeing another chiropractor but was limited to only one visit a month because that was all that my insurance company was willing to cover.

After coming to the office, I knew that I needed help as my health was failing. The information I received I knew would save my life.

My Health has improved 150%. I feel like new women inside and out. I'm able to swim and exercise at the gym. I'm able to walk without any pain and further than I was able to before. Plus, I sleep better and I can lie flat when I sleep. I'm telling everyone I know that chiropractic is life changing. God bless the doctors and staff at Champion Chiropractic. My power is turned on and there's no stopping me now!

-Maria F.
August 8, 2007

I had lower back pain, asthma, morning sickness (runny nose, sneezing, coughing and shortness of breath). I was never really informed about Chiropractic Care so I had no prior feelings. But I feel great about it now. Since coming to Champion Chiropractic I haven't had to take any medications. I have no more morning sickness and no more asthma attacks and my body weight was shifted to the left 20 pounds now it is only seven pounds. I would tell my family and friends that it is great and you definitely feel better.

-Sanjay B.
June 12, 2003

Before receiving Chiropractic care my doctors diagnosed me with Congestive Heart Failure. I could not breathe or sleep, because I was out of breath. I was recommended to Champion Chiropractic and after a few adjustments, I felt much better and more energetic than I had felt since I was first diagnosed by my doctors.

I was unaware about Chiropractic care and certainly did not understand how much alternative care would help me.

After my third adjustment, I am more confident that I have made the right decision in seeking alternative care. I feel much better and my heart is not racing anymore. I can breathe better than the doctors ever thought I would be able to. I don't need my pacemaker and my heart is strong. I strongly recommend Chiropractic care to everyone.

My health and my quality of life is improved beyond my expectations. My co-workers cannot believe the difference in my health and how quickly I was able to come back to work.

I do not need my heart monitor anymore. I want to spread the word to others about my experience and results.

I have told all of my friends and co-workers how this experience has changed my life. I feel better, stronger and healthier than I have felt since I have trusted and believed in Chiropractic care.

-Sharon J.,
February 21, 2008

⌣⌣⌣

Before receiving Chiropractic care, I had constant sinus attacks and stuffiness; I was having severe menstrual cramps, numbness and tingling in the feet when I walked. I knew the positive effects of Chiropractic care, but had no idea that it dealt with the entire body. I thought it was mainly for accident victims, not for "well" people, therefore I was skeptical. I was so overwhelmed at the wealth of information available on nutrition, exercise, total man and the relationship between Chiropractic care and the overall functions of your body. My sinus attacks have stopped and I have more energy, less intense and frequency of menstrual cramps and I have even improved my diet. I am able to focus better and being in a very high stressed job such as nursing this is important. I am also able to balance all tasks and have achieved multiple other positive results. Chiropractors are special people and they can tap into your physical as well as your spiritual being. Without Chiropractic care your body can be out of balance. "I urge everyone to try it, you won't regret it.

-Vivia W.
12/06/2004

❧❧❧

Before receiving chiropractic care I was always having back, shoulder &heel pain sometimes it was so painful to move my arms, bend over, and even get out of bed. My back hurts so badly at night that I would always have to use those over the counter drugs to get relief, I could not walk in the mornings because of the pain in my heel.

Chiropractic care always made sense to me but I never went to one as I thought the pain I was feeling was only from a strained muscle in my back and shoulder or from my improper bending or lifting incorrectly.

After being introduced to Dr. Yachter and he showed me my first X-ray he explained things to me about treatment, I started to have hope that I'll be free from pain. I started getting my adjustments, which I look forward to. The pain in my heel is gone. I'm having less back and shoulder pain and now I'm starting to get lots of energy. The next X-ray I took showed so much improvement that gave me will power to continue with my treatment. I realized my entire health and quality of life was improving. Since beginning care I stop using the back rub creams and over the counter drugs.

I'm very thankful for the treatments I received but most of all I'm thankful for the education I've received at Champion Chiropractic's Power Workshops.

I would encourage everyone to get X-rayed to find out how to get his or her bodies the way God designed it to be.

Last but not least the staff at the Champion Chiropractic office is very nice. They make everyone feel at home when you go there. It's just like one big happy family together. Thanks to Dr. Yachter and his staff, you guys are the best. GOD BLESS!!!!!!!!!!!!!!!!!!!!!!!!!!!!!!!!!

-Winsome A.,
2/13/2004

᷍᷍᷍

Before receiving Chiropractic care I was in constant chronic pain. My entire body ached and it was painful to move my head, or to accomplish simple tasks such as writing letters or reading books.

The mattress that I had made it very painful when I went to sleep, and also caused excruciating pain to my back. This also caused me to constantly having to take over the counter drugs.

Chiropractic care always made sense to me, but not many people I knew went to one so I didn't either. I didn't think it was for me because of my circumstances. However, after Dr. Yachter explained the causes of my condition and the treatment that I needed, I felt hopeful that I no longer had to live in pain. I look forward to my adjustments and realized that my entire health and quality of life was going to improve.

Since beginning my care I have stopped taking over the counter drugs for pain, I have learnt the horrible effects that drugs can have on your body. I am thankful for the treatments here, but more importantly I am thankful for the education I've received at Champion Chiropractic.

I truly encourage people to get x-rayed, find out how to get well the way that God created our bodies to heal. It is the only way for His power to be released in our bodies for perfect wellness. You won't be sorry you began on the road to "GOOD HEALTH".

-Yvonne S.,
2003

ᴊᴊᴊ

When I was a teenager, I hurt my lower back by lifting something incorrectly. I was told by the doctor that I would always have problems. I also suffer daily with headaches, pain and mitral valve prolapse. I was told by my doctor I would most likely have heart failure in the future.

We are so trained by the world and the medical fields, that I always believed chiropractors were quacks and not real doctors.

After the seminars in my church and the orientation here, I was just blown away by the lies I have been told.

As of today, I might have a headache once every two weeks and it does not stop me from functioning as before. About three weeks into my care, I had a week of tests that normally would throw me into deep depression and most likely several angry outbursts. The most unbelievable peace came over me that week. I did not react and it feels great. The calmness continues today.

Please don't believe what we have been trained to believe. Research and gain the knowledge for yourself. It has changed my life. There were so many things I did not know before the seminars about my care. God says without knowledge my people will perish.

Power is ON! God Bless!

-Brenda B.,
November 2, 2006

Prior to receiving care by Dr Yachter, I was in daily back pain due to severe scoliosis. I was having difficulty walking, sitting, and even sleeping. My blood pressure was higher than it had been in years and I was experiencing severe fatigue on a daily basis.

I had received Chiropractic care many years ago and found it to be very beneficial. However, due to my current health coverage, I was discouraged from seeing a Chiropractor even though traditional medicine had been unable to help me for years.

My experience with Champion Chiropractic was at once a positive one and reminded me that only through regular Chiropractic care could I receive any relief from my constant neck and back pain caused by severe scoliosis. But beyond that, I have learned so much more about the Central Nervous System, how it works and how valuable nutrition is to our over-all well being. The education has been invaluable.

Over the past several weeks, I have received many comments from family and friends telling me that I look better than I have in a long time, that I am walking much straighter and taller, not so crooked any more. I have more energy and stamina than I have had in the past two years. And my blood pressure is the lowest it's been in about three years!

I strongly suggest to family and friends the enormous value of seeking Chiropractic care. I would much rather find the source of the problem; take action to correct it, than to take medications to eliminate symptoms while doing possible long-term harm or damage to the body.

I am a strong advocate of Chiropractic care. The added value of the workshops and training provided through Champion Chiropractic show the total commitment of Dr Yachter and the entire staff. Thank you so much for caring about your patients.

-Joyce S.,
February 2, 2007

Before coming to chiropractic care, I was a mess. My back ached terrible, my sinuses were real bad, I constantly blew my nose and now all that is gone. I had tingling in my hands and fingers all the time. Now that's gone. I also had cramps in my legs, and that's gone. Thank God for chiropractic care.

Before I came to the chiropractor, to Dr. Yachter, I had been to a few chiropractors but they never gave me the information I got here. They just took x-rays and gave me massages, never explaining anything about the nerve system.

After coming here, to Champion Chiropractic, I was amazed to learn so much about the functions of the spinal column and the nervous system and what happens when it is not functioning right.

Now my health has improved tremendously since I began my care here, both physically and spiritually. I have a better attitude towards my health and a better understanding of my body.

I would tell anybody, friends and family members, they need to have themselves checked out, because life and death is in the power of the nerves and spinal cord which flows through our body.

-Mariette B.,
October 9, 2006

The health problems that affected my daily life were acid reflux, neck pain and lack of energy. I was afraid to eat certain foods, because of the acid reflux. I had many nights as to where I was sleepless. I didn't have energy to do many things like cook and help kids with homework because I felt tired and sleepy.

I thought chiropractors were just temporary and momentary doctors, which took away my pain for those 30 minutes.

After coming to the office, my feelings were that the doctor at Champion Chiropractic is here to heal the body through the spine, for a life time.

Now I have no acid reflux, I sleep 100% at night. I have more energy to do my daily activities and I feel like I am 100 pounds lighter.

This chiropractic office realigns the spine so that the body will and can be free of diseases or sicknesses they may have had in the past. Chiropractic corrects the incorrect curve in the neck and leads to a life- long of good health and a disease free body.

-Lolita B.,
October 10, 2006

∿∿∿

Before coming to Champion Chiropractic the health problems that affected my life were depression, anxiety, migraines, dizziness, stomach problems but most of all I wasn't able to get pregnant. I wasn't so sure chiropractic care could help me because I always thought you only saw a chiropractor after a car accident or slip and fall.

I am very thankful and pleased I did start seeing Dr. Yachter because I would have never became healthy and after starting care I was blessed with a beautiful healthy baby. Chiropractic care has made me stronger in every way.

I would tell all my friends and family that they need to come to Champion Chiropractic if they want to feel better and to get off medications.

-Zandra O.,
March 3, 2009

꒰꒰꒱꒱

Prior to chiropractic care, I had an indescribable pain in my stomach every night for about 3 to 4 hours causing me to spit up acid. After about 3 weeks of seeing Dr. Yachter I was able to sleep through the night with no pain.

Going to see a chiropractor never crossed my mind because I always thought chiropractors were just for victims of an accident. I never would of have thought that it would change my life but it has!

I love Dr. Yachter; my 7 year old son has even considered becoming a chiropractor after feeling the results of adjustments. It hasn't just changed my life but everyone in my life. My health has improved greatly improved; sleeping has now become an all night pleasure. Not having to endure the pain that I had is overwhelming!

I tell everyone I know you need to come in for an exam don't worry about the price, without having your health you'd have no life. It's miserable and impossible to enjoy living life in pain.

-Lisa W.,
January 14, 2009

Before receiving chiropractic care some of the health problems that affected my life were tightness in the right side of my neck, mid back and lower back. My vision was declining and I wasn't breathing as easy. As a professional athlete it made me feel slower and fatigued.

I was not educated in chiropractic care although I am very health conscious it helped me a lot. It has given me more energy, life, vitality, as well as having more power physically and breathing is much easier.

I would tell all my friends and family that seeking chiropractic care is a wise investment

-Luke Scott
March 2, 2009

About the Author

Dr. David Yachter is 1993 alumni of Life University and has maintained a full- time practice in Plantation, Florida since graduation. As a formally trained endurance athlete, his knowledge and experience in the realm of high performance health and healing has been instrumental in generating one of the largest clinics of its kind in the country. Dr. Yachter is responsible for leading and participating in numerous international healing mission trips and was awarded Chiropractor of the Year in 1998, 2006 and 2007. With more than 50 local and international speaking engagements annually, Dr. Yachter regularly helps local charities, clubs, business, and religious organizations by teaching healthy lifestyle workshops. He is married to Yvette Yachter and are both the proud parents of their three boys: Joshua, Leon, and Gavin. Dr. Yachter's passion for leading and inspiring his patients and peers continue to create transformational change in the lives he touches around the world.

EDUCATION
University of Florida, Gainesville, FL
Life University, Marietta, GA
Doctor of Chiropractic

LICENSURE
State of Georgia
State of Florida

ADVANCED TRAINING
- Exercise Physiology
- Nutrition
- Life Management Programs
- Sports Performance and Injury
- Maternity Care and Pediatrics
- Chiropractic Biophysics
- Pettibon Technique
- CLEAR Institute Non- Surgical Scoliosis Correction
- Physician Certification: Workers Compensation
- Elevation Health Regional Provider

PROFESSIONAL AFFILIATIONS
- International Chiropractors Association
- Florida Chiropractors Society, Past President
- Southern Chiropractic Association

NATIONAL SPEAKING ENGAGEMENTS
- Dynamic Essentials Seminars
- SCA Saturday Night Live
- Maximized Living Seminars

ACHIEVEMENTS AND HONORS

- Chiropractic Missions:
  1997: Panama City, Panama
  1998: Kingston, Jamaica
- 1998, 2006, 2007 CHIROPRACTOR OF THE YEAR
- 2000 BJ Palmer Service Award
- 2001, 2004 Tree of Life Award

HEALTH, INJURY & PERFORMANCE CONSULTING
- Miami Dolphins Pro Football
- Florida Marlins Pro Baseball
- Florida Power & Light (FPL)
- Nova Southeastern University Official Chiropractor
  Baseball Team
- Florida Bobcats Arena Football: Official
  Chiropractor
- Broward Community College: Swimming & Diving
  Teams
- American Airlines
- Delta Airlines
- SAMS Wholesale Club
- Department of Transportation: City of Ft.
  Lauderdale
- Nortel Communications
- BellSouth Communication
- Lowes Home Improvement
- Culligan Water
- Toys R Us
- Primerica Corporation

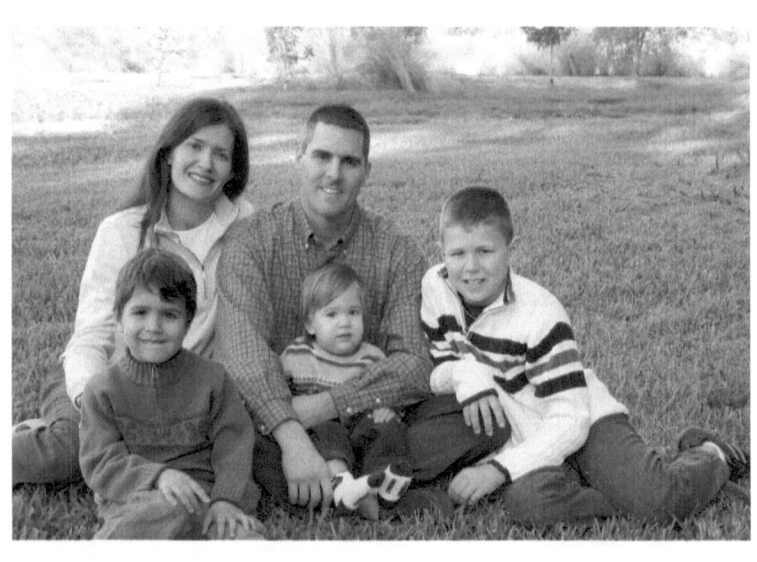

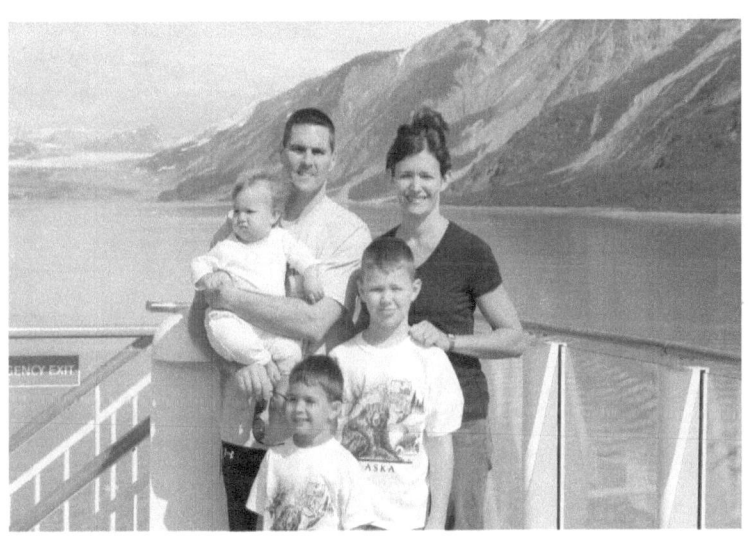

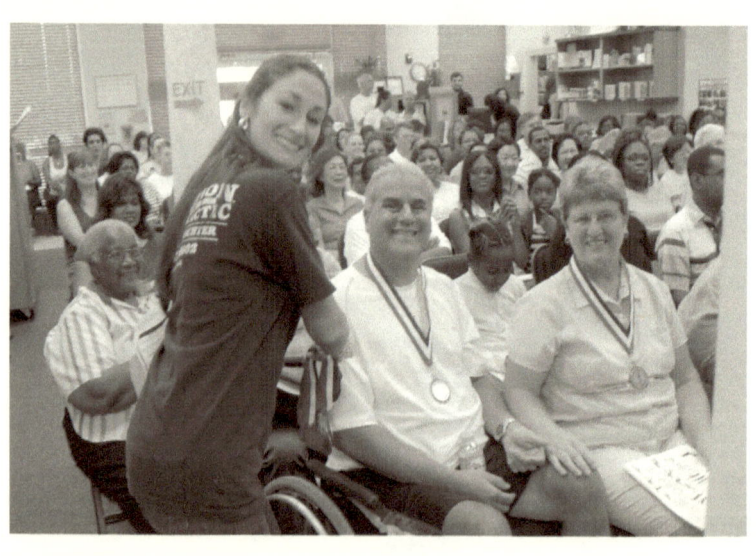

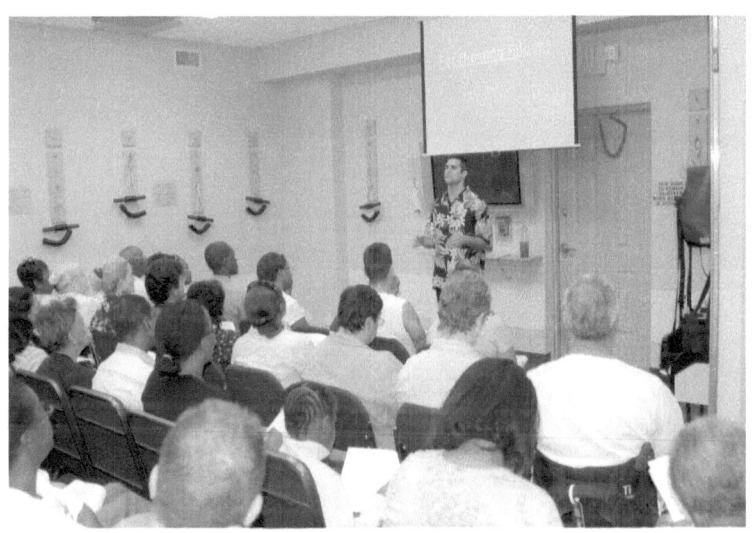

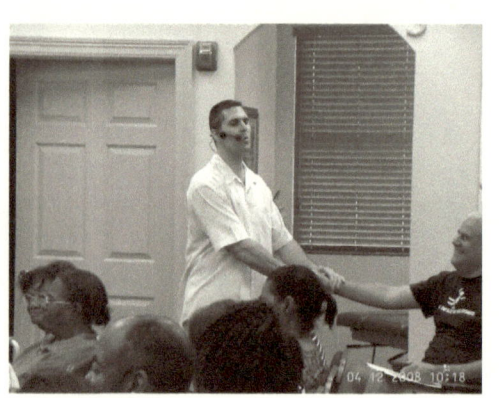

www.ingramcontent.com/pod-product-compliance
Lightning Source LLC
Chambersburg PA
CBHW031323290526
45784CB00014B/877